VITAL SIGNS

VITAL SIGNS

Heartbreaking, sometimes hilarious stories of a junior doctor's first year

IZZY LOMAX-SAWYERS

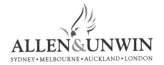

ALLEN&UNWIN
SYDNEY · MELBOURNE · AUCKLAND · LONDON

First published in 2022

Text © Isabelle Lomax-Sawyers, 2022

Allen & Unwin
Level 2, 10 College Hill, Freemans Bay
Auckland 1011, New Zealand
64 (9) 377 3800
auckland@allenandunwin.com
www.allenandunwin.co.nz

83 Alexander Street
Crows Nest NSW 2065, Australia
(61 2) 8425 0100

A catalogue record for this book is available from the National Library of New Zealand.

ISBN 978 1 98854 790 9

Design by Saskia Nicol
Set in Gotham
Printed and bound in Australia by Griffin Press

10 9 8 7 6 5 4 3 2 1

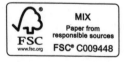

MIX
Paper from
responsible sources
FSC® C009448

The paper in this book is FSC® certified. FSC® promotes environmentally responsible, socially beneficial and economically viable management of the world's forests.

For Kyle

Author's note

As a doctor, it is my responsibility to keep patients' health information confidential. The stories contained within these pages have been written with anonymity and privacy in mind. The names of all patients and some staff and friends have been changed. Many identifying details have also been changed — this might include age, gender, ethnicity, occupation, nature of illness or, in the case of psychiatry patients, specific details of delusions. Many of the patients described are not 'real' people, although of course parts of their stories will ring true for some readers. Cases described in detail to illustrate how ward-round notes are written are purely fictional. Julia is not someone from my year of medical school, and her name and many details from her family's story have been changed.

Contents

CHAPTER 13

Beep

YOU'RE CARRYING A patient file, a ring binder packed full of clinical notepaper, ECGs, nursing care plans and discharge planning forms that threaten to fall out as you scribble your note. Between the synthetic scrubs and the N95 mask you're sweating like a pig. The boss is talking faster than you can write, your protective goggles are fogging up, you've needed to pee since five patients ago and it will be another hour until you can.

You're a first-year doctor at Middlemore Hospital in South Auckland, one of the busiest hospitals in New Zealand, and you're partway through a very long list of new patients to see on your morning ward round. Your phone rings for the fifth time in ten minutes. You hand the notes to the registrar to keep writing, and step outside the curtain to answer it. 'Kauri House Officer, Izzy speaking.'

Mark, a nurse from the Medical Assessment Unit in ED, wants to know if he can take a patient off cardiac monitoring. It's a new patient you've never met, and whom you know next to nothing about. 'Sorry, we haven't seen her yet. Can I let you know after?'

You slip back into the bedspace, where the boss is saying that this patient needs a CT scan. You quickly grab a laptop on a trolley to fire through an electronic order, then brace yourself to speak to the radiologist. You dial the operator, who accidentally puts you through to the CT bookings coordinator. You apologise, and dial again. This time, you get through.

'Hi, it's Izzy, one of the medical house officers. I'm calling to discuss a CT KUB request for Mr Andrews,' you say.

'Sure, let me read through the request.'

You wait nervously. Radiologists are the guardians of the hospital's limited available scanning slots, and they decide whether the benefit of the scan you requested is worth the radiation dose to the patient. This radiologist is renowned for being particular about request forms, and you did this form in about 30 seconds between patients. Your work phone starts to ring, but you decline the call. It rings again. 'Hi, can you ring back in five minutes?' you say to the nurse on the other end, and hang up, apologising to the radiologist.

'Have you done a urine?' the radiologist asks. You haven't, and you're desperate to, but she means the patient's urine. You should have put that information on the request form. 'Yes, sorry.' You read out the urinalysis result.

'Now, why do you want a CT KUB and not an ultrasound?' the radiologist asks. You have no idea. You offer to check with the team and call back. The boss says an ultrasound would be fine, so you call the radiologist to let her know. She changes the scan request to an ultrasound from her end, and you thank her.

The rest of the team is already with the next patient, Mrs Beauchamp. You join them, pulling the curtain behind you and waving at the patient. She's about your mum's age, and you admitted her the night before with a suspected TIA or mini-stroke. When she came in she had an irregular pulse, and her ECG showed an irregular heart rhythm called atrial fibrillation (AF), which can cause a stroke. Her heart is back in a normal rhythm now, but you suspect that it may have been flicking in and out of AF for a while. She'll need some investigations, including an ultrasound of the heart called an echocardiogram or 'echo'. She'll also need to be started on blood thinners to prevent a stroke, and will probably take them for the rest of her life.

She's terrified, and tearful. She's young in the grand scheme of things, healthy until now, other than a single medication for blood pressure, works a professional job and has children in their teens and early twenties. She'd expected that it would be years before she had to confront her mortality. The boss squeezes her hand and makes comforting noises. You nudge a box of tissues her way. Your phone rings. You give the notes to the reg and step outside.

'Kauri House Officer, Izzy speaking.'

It's the nurse who tried to call before. 'Hi, it's May from Ward 33 east. I'm just letting you know I'm sending Mr Chua to the discharge lounge.'

You thank her and hang up. The rest of the team are still comforting Mrs Beauchamp, and it is an awkward time to rejoin them. You find the file for the next patient on the list, Mr Donald, and start preparing the ward-round note as you wait outside the curtain. You read through what the admitting doctor has written overnight, and click through a few things on the computer. Then you grab a fresh piece of clinical notepaper and lay down the bones of a note.

CWR McNeill (Kauri)
45M
1) UGIB
2) EtOH excess

Vital Signs

S:

O/E: EWS=0 Hb 105

Imp:

Plan:
1. CIWA
2. NBM for OGD
3. Pabrinex
4. Cont omeprazole
5. Call if melaena, haematemesis, HR>110, SBP<100
   or concerns
6. Advise EtOH reduction

During your first clinical placements in medical school, these notes with their acronyms and jargon might as well have been in another language, but you now write like this without even thinking. CWR McNeill is the consultant on this ward round. The patient is a 45-year-old man whose problems are an upper gastrointestinal bleed, and alcohol (EtOH) intake in excess of recommended limits. As a junior doctor working in medicine (not psychiatry), it's not your place to label him with a diagnosis, but that it exceeds recommended limits is an objective fact. He has been drinking twelve beers every night for years, and more on weekends.

You've been on this rotation for a month, and already you know the patterns for how to treat the handful of problems responsible for most hospital admissions. Anyone who drinks as much as this man needs to be observed closely to make sure he isn't going into life-threatening alcohol withdrawal; the withdrawal scale used at this hospital is called CIWA, and you have never cared to learn what that stood for. He also needs Pabrinex, an intravenous multivitamin that replaces all the nutrients he's missed out on when drinking twelve beers a night hasn't left him with much appetite for food. People who drink this much for this long are at risk of irreversible brain damage, not so much from the alcohol directly, but from vitamin B1 or thiamine deficiency.

It's also your team's responsibility to give him what is called 'brief advice' that it would be a good idea for his health if he cut back on drinking.

He will need a camera down his throat to find and treat the cause of bleeding, and he will need intravenous antacid medication to speed up the healing of whatever has bled, and protect it from the powerful acid we all have in our stomachs. Bleeding in the upper gastrointestinal tract can be incredibly dangerous. You know doctors who have watched people bleed to death from it, vomiting blood faster than it could be replaced, and faster than they could get to the source of the bleeding to stop it.

You finish the note with your name and medical council number via a stamp that you wear on your lanyard, and you scribble your phone extension so the nurses can contact you. The boss has just finished with Mrs Beauchamp, and joins you and the registrar outside Mr Donald's room.

'Who do we have here?' asks the boss, and you quickly rattle off what you've read in the admission note.

> *Mr Donald is a 45-year-old man admitted following an episode of haematemesis yesterday afternoon. Sounds like he did also have an episode of melaena. No regular meds. He drinks twelve beers a night, no other medical history, no red flag symptoms. Works as a builder. Hb 105, haemodynamically stable. He has two IV lines and is consented and starved for OGD this afternoon. He's getting IV omeprazole and has Pabrinex charted.*

Vital Signs

The patient isn't in the bedspace when you walk in. The bathroom door is closed.

'Mr Donald?' the boss calls through the door. 'It's the doctors. Shall we come back in five minutes?'

You use the time to check blood results from the morning phlebotomy round. Mr Andrews has low potassium, so you chart him some potassium replacement. The phone rings. It's a nurse hoping you can chart an enema for a patient who hasn't had a poo in four days. You're happy to, but when you open the patient's electronic medication chart, she still has it open and you're locked out. Your registrar enters her password to override the nurse, and you prescribe the enema, along with two extra types of laxatives that the patient hasn't tried yet.

Back to blood results. A patient who has been in for a few days has had an improvement in his kidney function. You calculate his creatinine clearance and check the dose of a blood thinner he is on. He can now move up to a slightly higher dose. You check with the registrar that she's happy for you to chart it.

Mr Donald is out of the toilet now, and the team files back into his room. The boss greets him, and makes introductions. Your phone rings. You step out.

'Kauri House Officer, Izzy speaking.'

'Oh hi, it's Andrea calling from the discharge lounge. Just wanted to let you know that Mr Chua arrived.'

You thank her and hang up. The discharge lounge is a transitional lounge where people well enough for discharge from hospital can sit with a cup of tea and wait for their discharge papers or their ride home. It prevents beds from being taken up on the wards by people who no longer need them, often because the doctors are still rounding or attending to unwell patients, and are too busy to do the discharge papers. It's a good idea. It's also a major daily source of phone calls.

You rejoin the team, wheeling the laptop trolley with you. The boss is explaining the procedure Mr Donald will be getting that afternoon. 'It's a telescope that goes down the throat and looks in the food pipe or oesophagus, the stomach, and the first part of your small intestine. It can take photos of any sources of bleeding, but it can also be used to treat bleeds by burning or clipping small blood vessels. They can also take a biopsy if they see abnormal tissue. You'll be sedated, and you probably won't remember the procedure at all.'

The procedure isn't until the afternoon, so you prescribe some maintenance IV fluids to prevent dehydration. Your phone rings. 'Hi, it's Matt from Ward 1. Mrs East needs a vanc trough and the phlebs missed this morning. The dose is due now, could you please come and take her bloods?'

You finish charting the fluids, whisper to the reg where you're going, and hurry off to Ward 1. You stop at the staff toilets on the way, and finally, *finally* get to pee. You sit there in the quiet for a moment, eyes shut, scrubs around your ankles. Your phone rings. You let it go to voicemail.

You get to Ward 1 and collect the things you'll need to take bloods: disposable tourniquet, butterfly needle, vacutainer hub, green blood tube, alcohol swab, plaster. Mrs East is in isolation because she has a drug-resistant bacteria which has caused a skin infection (cellulitis). The antibiotic she is on, vancomycin, has a narrow window of opportunity before it is potentially toxic. It requires careful monitoring to ensure that it is at a level that will effectively treat infection without toxicity. It's a pain in the arse.

You put on the disposable yellow gown and blue nitrile gloves, and go in to greet Mrs East. 'Morning, just here to take a blood test. Sorry that we've had so many goes at it today!'

Mrs East is 80, little and frail. Between her delicate veins and the blood thinner she's on for a mechanical heart valve, she bruises like a champ, and already has a couple of impressive red-purple stains to show you where the phlebotomist tried to get blood. You tie the tourniquet as gently as possible, and watch her thin veins stand out against her thin forearm. Veins like these are nearly impossible to keep still, and tend to move away from the needle the moment it pierces the skin. You'll try them if you have to, but you'd rather not. You move up to gently press your finger in the antecubital fossa, the inside of the elbow. The vein there is plump, but it's where the phlebotomist tried, and you can feel a small haematoma from the earlier efforts. Better not.

Your phone rings in your pocket. You let it go to voicemail. It rings again. You sigh, apologise to Mrs East, loosen the tourniquet, throw your gloves in the bin, gel your hands, and retrieve your phone.

'Kauri House Officer, Izzy speaking.'

'Oh hi, it's Vanessa calling from Ward 2. I'm looking after Mr Folau and he told me that he usually takes ibuprofen, but there's none charted. Could you please chart it?'

Mr Folau has an acute kidney injury. You explain that his kidney function is still not back to normal, and he shouldn't take ibuprofen at the moment. You put your phone back in your pocket, gel your hands, put gloves on, and put the tourniquet back on Mrs East.

There is a vein on the side of her wrist that is bouncy and not too mobile. This is the cephalic vein. Often large, straight and superficial, it is sometimes nicknamed the 'house officer vein' (or 'houseman's vein' in ancient times before most house officers were women). It will often get you out of trouble when the faithful veins in the antecubital fossa have failed you, and Mrs East has a beauty. You work quickly, cleansing the skin with the alcohol swab, opening the packets you brought with you, attaching the hub to the butterfly, and preparing the plaster. You hold the vein as still as you can with your other hand.

'Sharp scratch!'

The blood flows easily, filling the tube. You remove the needle, apply the plaster, and direct Mrs East to put some gentle pressure on the area to reduce bruising. You put the needle into the sharps container, throw away your rubbish, and stick Mrs East's patient ID label to the tube. You take off your gown and gloves. Inside, the gloves are wet with sweat as they come off. Gross. You wash your hands with soap and water.

You fill out a lab form, stick a label on that, too, and put the form and blood tube in a specimen bag. You swipe into the medication room to use the Lamson.

The Lamson is a system of pneumatic tubes connecting every ward in the hospital. In cylindrical pods it transports blood samples from the wards to the lab, urgent medications from the pharmacy to the wards, and on occasion, pieces of paper to wards that the doctor is too busy or too lazy to walk to. On this particular morning, there are no empty pods waiting by the Lamson, and therefore no way for you to send this sample to the lab. You call to request more, and wait the three minutes it takes for one to arrive. You stuff the specimen bag in, twist the lid closed, and drop the pod into the opening at the top of the Lamson station, where it will wait to be sucked away to the lab.

You are just walking towards the exit when you hear the loud, persistent beep of the ward's emergency bell. You glance up at the call bell display. Room 8B. You follow the swarm of nurses responding to the call. You run through the principles of caring for a deteriorating patient in your head as you walk, like you do on the way to every emergency bell and resus call. A, B, C, D, E. Airway, breathing, circulation, disability, exposure.

Walking into Room 8B, you're confused at first. There are no patients in the room. Then you register what you are seeing: on the floor by the window, nurses are crouched over an unconscious man with a vomit stain on his gown, and a distinctly blue look about his lips. You force yourself to sound calm.

'Hi, I'm Izzy, and I'm one of the medical house officers. What's going on?'

Vital Signs

A healthcare assistant responds. 'I came in to offer him a cup of tea and I found him like this. I don't know what happened. I couldn't wake him up so I pushed the bell.'

'Okay, is anyone looking after this patient? Is he for full resus?'

Christine, a Filipina nurse you've worked with many times before, speaks. 'Mr George is my patient. He's on dialysis and is here for an infected fistula. He's not for CPR but is for 777s. Do you want me to put one out?'

'Um . . .'

The nurses look at you. Your face burns, and your ears ring. A, B, C, D, E. Fuck.

'I'll just assess him first.'

You take a deep breath, get down on the floor to open his airway, and check for breathing. He's not breathing. The basic life support you have rehearsed hundreds of times tells you that the next step is CPR, but he doesn't want that. Even if he did, it wouldn't help him. You feel for his carotid pulse, and there is none. His eyes are half open, his pupils fixed and dilated. This man is dead. He was probably dead for fifteen or twenty minutes before the staff found him.

'He's not breathing and he doesn't have a pulse. I think . . .'

'Do you want me to call a 777, doctor?' Christine repeats. She's referring to a medical emergency call, which will bring relevant staff to the room to assist.

'No thanks, Christine, he's dead,' says a voice authoritatively. It's the charge nurse, who has just arrived. Oh thank god. She has been a nurse for longer than you've been alive, and even though you already knew there was nothing you could do for this man, it's reassuring to hear her say it.

You stand up, and gel your hands.

'Thanks, everyone. Do you think maybe we could get him back onto the bed and put a fresh gown on? I'll give his medical team a call to do the paperwork and notify his family.'

You make your way to the nurses' station and check which

team was in charge of his care, find the number for his registrar in the phone book, and dial.

'Hi, it's Izzy, one of the medical house officers. I'm calling about your patient, Mr George. Is now an okay time?'

'Sure, what's up?'

'I responded to an emergency bell a few minutes ago. Mr George was found on the ground beside his bed, and unfortunately he had died. When you get a moment, do you think you could come and do the paperwork and let his family know?'

'God, that's awful news, I only saw him an hour ago. I'm on my way. Thank you for calling.'

You hang up, take a couple of deep breaths to try to calm your frazzled nerves, and send your reg a text asking where the team is now. They're with Miss Henare, a new patient who has been admitted with hyperthyroidism and a fast heart rate. You hurry back to find them. When you arrive, the boss is explaining to Miss Henare that she has been given propranolol, a beta blocker, to slow down her heart rate until her anti-thyroid medicine starts working. The dose of propranolol that was started the night before has brought her heart rate down to a safe level and she can come off monitoring, but it's still faster than the boss would like, and the dose needs to increase. The reg has been wheeling the laptop along, so you go to her medication chart and change the dose of propranolol. Your phone rings.

'Kauri House Officer, Izzy speaking.'

'Oh hey Iz, it's Stephen. Mr Iosefo's inhalers aren't charted, are you happy for me to do a telephone order?'

The clinical pharmacists review the medications of most patients who pass through the hospital. They check that everything the patient usually takes at home has been charted for them to take while in hospital. More than that, they check that everything prescribed is appropriate, still indicated, that monitoring requirements are up to date, and that there is no reason to change the dose. They save doctors from screwing up by picking up any obvious prescribing errors before the medicine can be given to the patient. They educate patients on new medicines they are being given, and print medication cards that explain in lay terms the purpose of each medication. And if you're really lucky, and your pharmacist is as good as Stephen, they will sometimes take a telephone order on your behalf, to be signed off later. They are a house officer's best friend.

You agree, grateful, and return to listening to the ward round. Miss Henare wants to know if the smart meter recently installed on her property had anything to do with her hyperthyroidism. The boss tells her there is no association, but she doesn't seem reassured. She asks about natural options instead of the medications we have prescribed. The boss explains that unfortunately there aren't any natural remedies that will safely bring down her heart rate and treat her hyperthyroidism. She asks for a copy of her test results to take to her naturopath, and you send them to the printer. Your phone rings.

'Kauri House Officer, Izzy speaking.'

'Hi there, Andrea again from the discharge lounge. Mr Chua is still waiting for his discharge papers.'

You take a deep breath before responding, forcing yourself to sound friendly and helpful.

'Oh I'm sorry, I'm just a bit busy at the moment; we are still on the ward round. We told him it would be after lunch, I think probably about 2 p.m.'

'Okay, thanks. I'll let him know.'

You hang up, and collect your printing.

Mrs Joseph is the last new patient to see. She is in hospital with a chest infection on a background of severe emphysema, what we call an infective exacerbation of COPD. She has been coughing up green gunk for days, and has started having fevers.

She needs antibiotics and oxygen. She also needs a COVID vaccine, although she's too sick to get one at the moment. The boss gently asks if she is planning to be vaccinated. Her children have seen things on Facebook that made them worried about the vaccine being an experimental treatment, and they don't want her to get it. She is now terrified of the vaccine, but also terrified of dying from COVID, which is a pretty likely outcome for her if she does get sick.

The boss offers to send one of the junior doctors back to talk to her later and answer any questions or concerns she has about the vaccine. You wave at Mrs Joseph and smile, trying to make the part of your face that is visible over the N95 look as reassuring as you can.

Your phone rings. You step out.

'Kauri House Officer, Izzy speaking.'

'Oh hi Izzy, it's Mark. I called you earlier about whether Miss Henare could come off the cardiac monitor, and I just wanted to check what the team decided.'

'Yes, that's fine, Mark. Thanks for calling to remind me!'

You've missed the rest of the plan for Mrs Joseph, and will need to ask the reg later.

'Coffee and run the list?' the boss asks. You smile gratefully, hurriedly log off the laptop and plug it in, before jogging to catch up with the team. The boss buys three flat whites, and you find an outdoor table at the staff cafeteria. You all take off your N95s. You're sure your face must mirror theirs, covered in indentations and pressure marks from the metal wire that fits the mask snug to the face. You sip your coffee. It's the closest thing you've had to breakfast.

On the table, your phone rings. Your reg grabs it, and answers for you. 'Kauri team, this is Amy speaking.' You give her a grateful look. 'Okay, is she symptomatic? What's the blood pressure? Have you done an ECG? Okay, thanks. If you could please get an ECG, I'll be there in a few minutes.'

Vital Signs

Mrs Beauchamp is back in fast atrial fibrillation, her heart rate well over a hundred. You quickly run through the list of patients to clarify the plan, and any urgent jobs that need to be done. Then you run through the list of old patients, whom the reg will see on her own.

'I'm in clinic this afternoon. Any problems, give me a call.' The boss goes off to her office, and the reg goes off to see Mrs Beauchamp. 'Do you mind getting started on some jobs while I do this? I'll give you a call when I'm done.'

You swig the rest of your coffee, put your mask on, gel your hands, and make your way to what is usually the quietest doctors' area in the hospital to get started on your tasks for the day. There are scans to be ordered, blood results to chase, patients to be discharged and laxatives to be charted. You stare at your patient list, plotting which tasks you need to do first.

Your phone rings.

CHAPTER 23

Beginnings

'THE NEXT STATION is Middlemore,' announces a cheerful recorded voice as the train begins to slow.

I give my friend Lauren an excited grin as we crowd onto the platform with all the other hospital workers.

Middlemore Hospital looms before us, a jumble of mismatched buildings of various ages and styles. A friendly security guard stands at the entrance. We've been told to show our student IDs, since we don't have staff IDs yet. The guard nods and waves us through.

'Follow the Rainbow Corridor,' the orientation email had said, and now I understand. The main route from one end of the hospital to the other is a corridor with walls adorned by rainbows. I am grateful that Lauren suggested we get the train together on the first day; she had placements at Middlemore as a medical student, and already knows her way around the sprawling campus.

She leads me past reception, a gift shop, a few cafes, a sushi shop, a Subway and a pharmacy, then up an inclining corridor to another building, past security and parking services, the immigration and Pasifika offices, all the way to the learning centre, Ko Awatea. The hospitals I trained at were much smaller, and definitely didn't have Subway. By comparison, Middlemore feels like a shopping mall.

We are very early, but a handful of other newly minted doctors are even earlier, and are sitting around drinking coffee and chatting about what they did in the short break between university ending and work starting. It's nine months into the COVID pandemic, so nobody travelled overseas as they might in a normal year, but a few people visited the South Island for the first time.

In other parts of the globe, new doctors are graduating early into hospitals full of more COVID patients than they can treat, and seeing horrors we cannot even imagine, but we are lucky. The biggest impact of the pandemic on us, aside from perhaps a week or two away from the hospitals during the strictest parts of lockdown, had been the cancellation of our overseas electives. I had planned a pilgrimage to Scotland, with six weeks to see the Shetland Islands where my granny grew up, and a month in Edinburgh to coincide with the Edinburgh Fringe. Instead, I had stayed in Dunedin, which is known as 'the Edinburgh of the South' but it wasn't quite the same.

We are starting our first jobs as doctors in a country that we think has eliminated COVID, and at orientation we aren't even wearing masks. We will spend many months of that first year working through Auckland's interminable lockdowns, and within the year we will all be looking after COVID patients, but we don't know that yet. As far as we are concerned, we are living in a post-pandemic world.

I don't really know many people other than Lauren, and a couple of classmates from Otago. Most of my new colleagues trained in Auckland. The Otago Medical School year finishes later, and my break was only one week. I spent it slowly making my way up to Auckland, stopping in to see family along the way, with my little grey Toyota Yaris packed to bursting with all of my worldly possessions. I drove up the North Island for the first time, making the trip from Wellington to Auckland in a day, and hitting the motorway during peak traffic.

I met Charlie, my partner, in Dunedin, but she had moved to Auckland shortly after. When the time came to decide where to apply for jobs, I had applied for Middlemore so that I could follow her to Auckland. I had already perfected the story over the last few months of being asked my plans for my first postgraduate year (PGY1).

'I'm going up to Auckland to work at Middlemore,' I would say cheerfully to the patient, doctor or family friend who was asking.

'Why Auckland?' they would ask with a mock shudder.

'I thought I'd started dating a policy analyst, but then she got into Auckland Medical School!'

Our orientation begins with a mihi whakatau, run by the kaumātua. After we are welcomed into the space and sing some waiata, we arrange the chairs to sit in a huge circle. We have been asked to prepare a short pepeha, sharing our name and where we are from. I stumble through my pepeha, my practice the night before no match for my stage fright. The kaumātua smiles encouragingly.

The first lecture we have as new doctors at Middlemore is about equity. People from the management team speak to us about the demographics of the local population, the health-equity challenges and opportunities, and about their hope and expectation that we will be committed to achieving equity in our time there, and our careers generally.

My eyes shine with excitement. Equity is the thing that has kept me wanting to be a doctor through the hardest parts of my six-year medical degree, and I am so glad to have chosen to work at a hospital where the managers care about it as much as I do.

Next is a scavenger hunt designed to show us around the sprawling campus. I absorb very little from that whirlwind tour of the hospital. It's a competition, and most of the other new doctors have been students at Middlemore at some point in their training, so can navigate around much faster than I can take it all in. I do manage to absorb the most important information from the tour: where to get the best coffee. Elixir will become the most important part of my daily routine, and within a few weeks the staff will know my name and coffee order without having to ask.

The rest of orientation is more serious, with IT training, talks from specialist nurses and pharmacists, and tips from some house officers a year ahead of us who were in our shoes not so long ago. I try to absorb as much as I can, but it is a blur. I am so excited about starting that I could burst, and so nervous that I could spew.

Perhaps the most exciting part of all is free lunch. This is the best perk of being a junior doctor. We don't have protected lunch breaks, and carry a phone or pager to lunch with us every day. If there is a call, we have to answer it. If there is an emergency, we have to leave our lunch and attend it. In exchange, the hospitals feed us. Every so often when our contracts are up for bargaining, the employer suggests taking away free meals and replacing them with a small meal allowance, but so far the unions have managed to resist. They know that the free meals are the only reason any of us take a lunch break.

Armed with our new staff meal cards, we strut into the packed cafeteria. Some join the queue for the hot meals, while I make a beeline for the fridge to grab sushi (free sushi!) and yoghurt. And cheese and crackers, and some nuts, and a brownie just in case.

This cafeteria is where I will spend any brief moments of downtime in my 60-hour weeks. It is where I will glow a little bit when the lunch lady calls me 'Bubba', even though she calls everyone that. It is where I will get to know my colleagues, and where they will eventually become my friends.

Every medical drama needs a cast of characters, a ragtag assortment of doctors from different walks of life who are sometimes rivals but always comrades. For fans of *Grey's Anatomy* it is Meredith, Cristina, George and (Katherine Heigl's) Izzie eating lunch on gurneys in a quiet corridor. For fans of *Scrubs*, it is JD and Elliot vying for Dr Cox's approval on internal medicine ward rounds, while Turk is off cutting people open and trying to woo nurse Carla. For cynical misanthropes, it is Greg House insulting his team and defying Cuddy while chucking back painkillers like Skittles. (If you recognise none of these references, congratulations on your normal and balanced life. If you are like me and have faithfully binged all of these shows several times over and then run out of medical dramas, may I suggest doing what I did next and coming to medical school.)

In my story it is Brittany, Sam, Gaby and me, dressed in scrubs at an outdoor table, drinking flat whites in the sun, our phone ringtones standing in for a theme tune.

Sam is about my age, Māori, a former postgraduate student in plant biology before he made the jump to humans. We bonded over politics, being gay, and a shared rage at the injustices doctors see every day in an unequal society.

Brittany and Gaby are 24, often confused for one another by nurses, and in considering how to describe them both here I guess I can understand why. They are alike in the same way a cucumber is like a courgette. They are both tall, blonde, beautiful and impeccably dressed. They are both clever, kind and competent doctors. They are both planning to be surgeons when they grow up. And yet they are somehow not at all alike.

Vital Signs

Brittany is Reese Witherspoon to Gaby's Scarlett Johansson. Brittany is goofy dad jokes and gentle teasing, while Gaby is savage wit. I like them both immediately.

The three of them were friends in medical school, and all flatted together, but it was the mysteries of our hospital's team allocations that brought them to me, first working on the same psychiatric ward as Brittany, and then joining the same orthopaedic team as Sam and Gaby. They will become the people I celebrate with when one of us learns a new skill or gets told we've done a good job, and the people I vent with when the computer system is down and the paperwork is piling up, or when a short and simple task has been interrupted by twenty phone calls.

Each one of us has an origin story, the radioactive spider bite or vat of nuclear waste that led us to give up our twenties in pursuit of a 60-hour work week in synthetic drawstring pants.

My origin story has been asked for and told so often that it has almost become a myth.

I left high school when I was sixteen, and moved cities to live with a boyfriend. I had been a bright but poorly engaged pupil, and I hadn't stayed at school long enough to gain university entrance. I spent a few years working in an administrative job, and convinced the local university to let me do some part-time study. My relationship with my boyfriend wasn't a particularly happy one, and I spent a lot of time bingeing box sets of *Grey's Anatomy* and *House*.

Those shows sparked my interest in medicine. I loved the puzzles, the drama, and how important and meaningful every-thing seemed. For a little while, I looked seriously into the prospect of studying medicine. I researched which high-school science subjects I would need to catch up on to give myself a better chance of getting in. I made a shortlist of halls of residence I could stay at in Dunedin. I watched the documentary *Donated to Science*, about Dunedin medical students dissecting cadavers, and imagined myself walking those hallowed halls and thinking deep existential thoughts in a white lab coat. I told my boyfriend about this half-a-plan. He didn't want to move, and I suppose I wasn't ready to leave him, so that was that.

Bored in my job, I decided to give full-time study a go, and after dabbling in various social sciences for the first year of university I ended up majoring in linguistics. I got involved in political and environmental groups on campus. I moved to Wellington to be closer to my family, and partway through my degree I got the opportunity to work at Parliament as an executive assistant for a Green politician. I took the job and put my studies on hold for a while. It was interesting work, and it was work I could throw myself into, but ultimately it was another administrative job.

A couple of years into the job I turned 22. At the time, 22 felt altogether too old to have no degree and no idea what to do with my life. I felt very insecure about not having finished university, and was worried that I would waste my potential. I returned to my studies part time. I tried out first-year law, but it was tiring and difficult, and four extra years to complete law school felt like too much study. After that I was three papers away from finishing my Bachelor of Arts, which would mean at least having a degree. I chose a few linguistics papers and knuckled down.

My 'last ever day of university' was a Wednesday in June. The wind whipped down Kelburn Parade and blew my hair into my eyes as I waited at the bus stop. My hands were covered in smudges of blue ink, the outside of my right pinky finger paper-burned from three hours of scribbling. To pass the time waiting for the bus, I called my mum.

'Hey, guess what?'

'What, darling?'

'I'm done with university forever! No more exams!'

Vital Signs

I smiled at the grey sky.

'Very good, darling,' said Mum, not really picking up what I was putting down. 'Now, I've been looking into medical school. You can get in based on any undergraduate degree, so I think you should do that.'

I scoffed. Her suggestion was completely out of the blue, and ridiculous. I had only just managed to convince myself to go back to uni to finish the last six months of my BA. No way was I signing up to study for six more years!

'Being a doctor sounds like a boring job,' said my dad, a lawyer.

'Nah, you shouldn't do it. You won't finish studying till you're 30! That's really old!' said my best friend, Wilbur.

A month later I was submitting my application.

I can come up with plenty of good reasons why I did it. I like working with my hands as well as my brain. I enjoy working with people. My favourite jobs are ones that are busy but rewarding. I hate being tied to a desk. Probably these are all true reasons why I went to medical school, but the truest reason was a *Grey's Anatomy* box set at sixteen.

Gaby has always known a lot of doctors. Her mum is a GP, and a lot of her family friends growing up were in medicine. She has always admired medicine as a profession, but for most of her school years she didn't really consider becoming a doctor herself.

That changed when Gaby was fifteen and her mum was diagnosed with cancer. Gaby and her family spent a lot of time in and out of hospital as her mum received treatment, and was eventually cured. Gaby sees that as her origin story, the start of a slow realisation that she wanted to make a difference for others, the way her mum's medical team had done in her life. It wasn't a light-bulb moment, but it made her see medicine as an option. Later on, when it came time to make decisions about her career path, becoming a doctor felt like a happy marriage of the science subjects she was good at, and working with people which she enjoyed. She enrolled in biomedical sciences first year at Auckland, and got into medical school first try.

Sam knew from the start of high school that he wanted to be a doctor. He wanted to help people, but like a lot of young people he also really wanted to get out of the small town where he grew up. He also knew he was gay, and he thinks part of him hoped that if he pursued an impressive career, everyone would be proud of him even when he came out. He planned his high-school subjects around the sciences and mathematics he knew he would need to get into medical school. When he finally left his poor rural high school to go to university, though, he found he had to compete with the rich private-school kids whose education had carefully prepared them to succeed in competitive university courses. He tried his best in the first-year pre-med course, but didn't manage to get into medicine. He decided he was 'too dumb' to be a doctor, and gave up on his dream.

He knew he enjoyed science, so he decided to keep going with a science degree. He finished his undergraduate degree in biology, and even did a Master's. Then he took some time to travel and figure out what to do next. He took a job in South Korea teaching English, which was fun until it wasn't. He needed another change, and he decided to give medicine one more go. He figured he had nothing to lose by putting his hat in the ring, and if it didn't work out, he could continue his science studies and do a PhD. He put in an application and was accepted.

Brittany didn't really know what she wanted to do with her life when she was in school, but she thought that medicine seemed like an interesting and challenging thing to study, so she decided to see if she could get in. She was clever and worked hard, and when she was offered a place in medical school she decided to accept it. It was only when she did her first surgical placement that she knew for sure that she was supposed to be a doctor.

My girlfriend, Charlie, is a medical student. When she was in high school she wanted to be a doctor, but she managed to fail chemistry, physics and maths, all of which would be part of the competitive first year that decides entry to medical school. Although she never really stopped wanting to be a doctor, she stopped expecting that she would be able to.

She persevered through a double degree in sociology and law, and the more she learned about the inequities that make some people's lives shorter and harder, the more her passion grew for health. She also fell in love with *Call the Midwife*, and the idea of having a vocation.

After she finished university, she didn't know what she wanted to do. She was burnt out and exhausted from study, and feeling less than inspired by the idea of going straight into a job in an office. She decided to take a gap year and travel. She lived in Spain, and worked part time as a waitress. She spent most of her free time taking long walks through the European countryside, contemplating what she would do next. On one of these long walks, it came to her that life was too short. She had to follow her heart and pursue medicine.

When it came time to return to New Zealand, and she started an office job, she did it alongside some postgraduate study in public health. She asked a medical student she followed on social media for advice about the application process. I was happy to chat, and answered her questions as best I could.

She got a job as a policy analyst in Dunedin, where I was studying at the time. She didn't really know anyone, so I suggested meeting up for a coffee so I could show her around. She applied to both Auckland and Otago medical schools, not really daring to hope that she would get a place right away.

We became fast friends, and I think it was probably when I

made my friend Amber drive me to Charlie's house to drop off a block of chocolate after she'd had a bad day that I realised I had a bit of a crush on her. I plucked up all my courage to tell her that I liked her, and as luck would have it, she liked me too.

We were just starting to think about dating when to her great surprise she was accepted into the medical programme at the University of Auckland. I had another two years of studying in the South Island, and we hadn't known each other for very long at all, so we knew it didn't make sense to try to do long distance. We had a tearful (on my part) trip to Dunedin airport, and said goodbye forever. Which of course was how, nearly three years later, I found myself in Auckland, living in a beautiful old house in Grafton called 'La Roche', a stone's throw from the medical school.

Our flatmate Āria is in medical school, a year behind Charlie. Like us, she came to medicine a little bit later on.

Āria spent a lot of time around doctors as a child. She herself had asthma and eczema in childhood, needed grommets for glue ear, had a childhood hip injury called a slipped upper femoral epiphysis (SUFE), which needed years of orthopaedic follow-up, and she got very sick with encephalitis as a teenager.

Āria's grandma was also very unwell for most of Āria's childhood. She had type 1 diabetes, as well as a mental illness for which she had several long periods of hospitalisation.

I think if you spend a lot of time in hospitals, you find being at a hospital either very traumatising or very comforting. For Āria, it was the latter. She liked hospitals, and they made her feel very safe. Like me, she became a fan of medical dramas. First it was *ER*, which she watched with her mum, and she had crushes on nurse Carol and nurse Abby (who later became Dr Abby). Then it was *Grey's Anatomy*.

In high school, she thought she might like to be a psychologist. She enjoyed talking to people and hearing about their problems, and wanted to help people. When it came time to decide whether to do science or art subjects in senior school, she chose history and English, because she was good at them and found them interesting. She knew she wanted to do a double degree at university, and her high-school boyfriend was going to law school, so she applied for a law scholarship and, to her surprise, she got it.

She went to university and studied law and history. She enjoyed it, and she was good at it. Her scholarship was sponsored by a law firm, and came with the opportunity for a graduate job as a lawyer, which she accepted. Before starting work, she did a gap year, working for an NGO in Tanzania. Part of her job there was working in sexual health, which she enjoyed immensely.

She came back to New Zealand ready to start her job as a lawyer. For five years she worked her way up, mostly doing corporate litigation. She found it interesting and stimulating work, but at the same time she felt increasingly aware that her career would keep her immersed in the corporate Pākehā world. The more senior she became, the greater the desire she felt to be doing work that served the community, and especially her Māori community.

When people had asked her what she would do if she wasn't a lawyer she had always said she would have been a doctor, but it had never seriously felt like a possibility. She had dropped the sciences in the latter years of high school, and didn't think she could realistically pick them up again. But in her last couple of years as a lawyer she met more and more people who did go back to medical school. A close friend returned from overseas and started studying medicine. A lawyer a few years ahead of her at her firm decided to become a doctor. It felt a little bit like the universe was letting her know it was possible.

Close to the time that she would need to have her application in, she worked with clients who were immersed in te ao Māori, the Māori world, and it cemented for her that investing in her cultural journey and serving her Māori community was something that she needed to do. She decided to apply to do pre-med. The law would still be there if it didn't work out, and she knew she could still have a satisfying career as a lawyer, but she felt she owed it to herself to see if she could be a doctor. She got in, and now works as a tutor for Māori and Pasifika pre-medical students embarking on the same journey.

Every medical student has their own wind in their sails, their own 'why' that keeps them at the library until closing time, and that propels them through six long years of study until the day they start work as doctors. We come to medicine from different backgrounds and for different reasons, but we all end up in the same place.

The night before my first day at Middlemore, my flatmates and I watched the first episode of *Grey's Anatomy*. It had been six years since I finally decided to pursue my dream and become a doctor, and twice that long since I had first watched Dr Webber tell the Seattle Grace interns that their years as surgical residents would be the best and worst of their lives.

I didn't know exactly what was ahead of me as a doctor, and I didn't know if it would be the best time of my life or the worst, but I was excited to finally start. Stepping off a train in Ōtāhuhu and striding down the Rainbow Corridor to get to the psych ward in time for handover, I knew it was time for the hard work to begin.

CHAPTER 3:

Madness

AS A TEENAGER I was prone to bouts of sadness — weeks or months when my emotions were too big to fit in my head and would leak out through my eyes. That is the idea I used to have of mental health: a sad teenage girl sitting with her back against a wall, hugging her knees and crying off her black eye make-up. I used to imagine psychiatric hospitals to be farmhouses in the countryside where people with big feelings could take a holiday from their lives to take long walks in the fresh air and write bad poetry.

That changed in my early twenties, when my friend Hermione was admitted to a psychiatric ward after a suicide attempt. It was the first time I had seen someone with depression so severe that it stole the ability to eat, shower and sometimes even speak. I would visit her as often as I could, and when I did she was always in the same spot, sitting on the end of her bed in dirty clothes with dirty hair, staring at nothing in particular.

Most visits I would stop by the Wishbone cafe to buy her

a coffee, one of the few things that still seemed to give her any enjoyment. I would yap at her with updates about my life, and ask her questions, which she often answered many seconds later, as if finally summoning the energy to speak. I later learned that her depression had come with a dose of psychosis — she would hear things that weren't really there, and receive messages from the universe in books. I wonder if I would have been able to tell that, if I'd had the training then that I've received since.

The locked psych ward was a frightening place for a fairly sheltered young woman like Hermione. It was full of older men whose illnesses made them disinhibited and not very good with boundaries, and people in the grips of psychosis who were unpredictable and sometimes violent. Hermione was physically assaulted by a fellow patient, and watched other patients assaulting staff and getting forcibly sedated with injections in the bum.

But people who are unwell usually pose a much greater risk to themselves than to anyone else. A few weeks after Hermione was hospitalised, a young man escaped from her ward by climbing the high wall that enclosed the courtyard, and was tragically found dead later that day. Hermione herself managed to escape from the locked unit several times in the months she was there, and the police were called to help find her. She was always found before anything terrible happened.

Some of the nurses were kind to her, even maternal, but a few seemed to have been broken by decades of being insulted and assaulted every day at work, making them petty, uncompromising and devoid of compassion.

If you ask Hermione now, years on, she will tell you that the mental-health system saved her life. She will also tell you that it left her with scars that may never fully heal. On one admission to hospital, she was put in a seclusion room entirely naked so that she couldn't hang herself with her clothes. She was given electroconvulsive therapy (ECT), sometimes known as shock therapy, against her will. This was life-saving, and was the only thing that helped when she was at her most unwell, but a side effect is memory loss, and she has forgotten most of a year.

Eventually, with the right combination of ECT and medication, her mental health stabilised enough that she didn't need to be in hospital anymore. She moved cities for university, and a fresh start. She worked hard to stay well. Her new psychiatrist and community psych nurses were excellent, and the group programmes she was enrolled in seemed to help.

Perhaps what helped most of all was that she was white and upper middle class, with a dedicated and financially comfortable family. Those privileges afforded her the opportunity many long-term psychiatric patients miss, of moving on with her life and leaving mental illness behind. She got a degree, and when she graduated she was offered a good job. When I see her now, she is dressed in designer clothes and talking in her fast and animated way about work, flatting and dating. Sometimes I can forget all about the version of her who sat still and silent in a hospital gown in that dreary little room.

When I found out that my first full run as a house officer would be in psychiatry, I tried desperately to get out of it. I advertised for a swap on the junior doctor Facebook group, and was met with laugh reacts (psychiatry is not a popular run) and the occasional reassurance that it wasn't a bad job. My reluctance to work in mental health wasn't out of a lack of love for patients in need of mental health services. I feel passionately about the need for a robust, compassionate mental health system with patients and whānau at the centre. I was just afraid that I would be working with the kinds of people who were unkind to Hermione. I was afraid that as a part of the system I would be privy to cruel comments, eye-rolling and stigma.

But despite my best efforts, I didn't manage to convince

anyone to swap with me, and so I started as a house officer at Tiaho Mai. It was a gentle introduction to doctor life. We had a late start as far as medical rosters go, the day beginning at 8.30 a.m. with a handover meeting. Whaea Ruby, the kuia, would open each meeting with a karakia, and sometimes we sang a song. Then the charge nurse would list each patient on the ward and tell us how their night had been. There were usually one or two new patients, and we would go through their psychiatric history and the reason they were in hospital. Brittany and I took turns typing a brief record of what had been discussed to put into the patients' electronic notes. About twenty minutes into handover, the patients from the locked ward would be taken to use the gym and basketball court. They would walk past the handover room, wave to us through the window or bang on the door.

After handover, the team made our way onto the ward to start meeting with patients. While I was at medical school I did some placements in more traditional psychiatric wards — dated buildings with comically large old-fashioned keys that the staff carried to lock and unlock rooms. Tiaho Mai is a psychiatric unit unlike any I had ever seen. Brand new and having recently won an architecture prize, its wards are laid out around a huge, sunny internal courtyard. It is nicer than any house I have lived in. A wharenui at the front provides a space for the kuia and kaumātua to welcome new patients. There is a gym, a basketball hoop, a ping-pong table, and a staff of occupational therapists who organise activities from painting to karaoke.

The psychiatrist on my ward was Kurt, who turned out to be the type of psychiatrist I would want to look after me if ever I needed it. He was thoughtful and kind to patients, and generous to a fault with his juniors. I don't think we paid for a single coffee in that three-month run, and at the end he took the whole team out for dinner. Working under him was a psychiatric doctor called Khalid, a gentle and compassionate man who drank a can of cold-brew coffee every morning, and had a soft spot for the 'naughty boys' under our care. He could sit with a young man in the grips of psychosis and make him feel safe and understood.

The psychiatric registrar, training to do Kurt's job, had a broad smile and a broader Aussie accent. She was one of the funniest people I've ever met, and is responsible for my favourite night-shift story of all time.

The psychiatric unit has a pull-out couch upstairs in the office area, which night staff can use to sleep on when things are quiet. On one set of night shifts there had been a lull in the stream of referrals from ED, and the registrar had gone upstairs to have a nap. She's normally a rubbish sleeper, but by some miracle she managed to grab a couple of hours of restful sleep before waking up needing to pee. So comfortable was her nap that she had somehow managed to kick off her scrub pants, and was in her top and underwear. It was three in the morning and nobody was around, so she didn't bother to put her pants back on when she toddled off to the bathroom.

The toilets were in the corridor outside the main office. It was only on her way back that she realised her mistake: the office had swipe-card access, and her swipe card was in the pocket of her scrub pants, along with her phone.

She had no choice but to walk downstairs to the only other part of the complex she could access without a swipe card: the reception desk. She sat behind the desk in her scrub top and undies, and called hospital security.

When the security guard arrived, he looked her up and down. 'So it's three in the morning and I'm at the psych ward, and you're not wearing pants. How do I know you're a doctor here and not a patient?'

He escorted her upstairs, where she could retrieve her pants and a little bit of her dignity, and show him the offending ID card.

'All right, Doc,' he said. Then he paused. 'You know, I've been doing this job for twenty years, and you would think I had seen it all. But I haven't seen this.'

In a psychiatric interview you try to elicit information by encouraging your subject to share what is going on inside their head. What they are actually saying tells you some of what you need to know. What is their understanding of why they are in hospital? How have they been feeling recently? Have they been worried that people are out to get them? Do they see or hear things that other people can't? Are they thinking about harming themselves, or someone else? Do they use alcohol or other drugs?

The rest of what you need to know comes from making observations about their appearance, thinking and behaviour. Are they in a ball gown and eight-inch heels at 9 a.m., or dirty trackpants and a hoodie? Do they seem to have showered, and is their hair clean? Is their speech fast, words spilling out of them all at once, or do they sit in silence for a long time when asked a question? Does what they are saying make sense, or are the connections between thoughts loose and hard to follow? Are they talking to entities that aren't really there?

For our Māori patients, Whaea Ruby would sit in on the interviews. She would help to make the ward interview rooms feel like warm and safe places. For Samoan patients, the social worker, Iliganoa, would often join the interview. I only ever met one patient who didn't want Iliganoa to be involved in their care, giving the reason that she was too in love with her. We could all see where she was coming from.

Our team looked after patients in the High Dependency Unit (HDU), a unit that was locked to keep patients safe and contained. Most of our patients (or 'service users' as they are sometimes known in mental health) were sectioned under the Mental Health Act, meaning that there was so much concern about their well-being and safety that they were legally required to stay in the hospital for a period of assessment and treatment by the psychiatrists. This was because a flare of their illness had made them a risk to themselves, others, or both. Two of the most common reasons for this were mania and psychosis.

Mania is an abnormal mood state seen in Bipolar Affective Disorder. A person suffering from mania is very elevated and often irritable. They are typically grandiose, may be flamboyant in clothing and manner, and cycle through topics and ideas at a breakneck pace that is nearly impossible to follow. Mania is a dangerous state to be in. Feeling invincible is not particularly conducive to self-preservation. People take extreme risks while manic — they might spend thousands of dollars they don't have, buy property they can't afford, take sexual risks they normally wouldn't, drive too fast or jump off tall buildings trying to fly. Some people in the grips of a manic episode have even bought and boarded flights overseas, ending up thousands of kilometres from home. Many people with bipolar disorder have a complicated relationship with mania, or hypomania (which is basically a milder version). While manic, senses are heightened, colours look brighter, and there is a sense of energy and elation. Some people describe it as the most alive they ever feel.

In contrast, for most patients, psychosis is a very frightening state to be in. Psychosis is basically a break from reality. We often associate it with the schizophrenia spectrum, but it can be seen in bipolar disorder, certain types of severe depression, or in people with vulnerable brains after taking recreational drugs. During a psychotic episode, people usually have some combination of delusions — false beliefs that they are totally convinced are true — and hallucinations. Their speech and thinking might be disorganised and chaotic. They are often paranoid and suspicious. They might be observed interacting with what we call 'non-apparent stimuli' — having conversations with someone nobody else in the room can hear, reaching for things that aren't there, or looking at things that nobody else can see.

A common delusion among people with psychosis is believing other people are reading or stealing their thoughts, or that their thoughts have been inserted by someone else. People commonly feel that they are being watched or followed, or that the government or gang members are out to get them, have been in the house, or have threatened them.

Sometimes, what we thought was delusion turns out to be reality. One young man, deep in a psychotic episode, kept telling us he was expecting a baby. This is a common delusion (although more so for women), and seemed unlikely for a whole host of reasons. When his mum visited for a family meeting, she told us that her son was hoping to come home in time for when his girlfriend gave birth.

One patient believed, or at least said, that she was married to Harry Styles and that they had five children. If she looked sad and someone asked what was wrong, she would explain that she and Harry had had a fight. She would agree to take her medicine or let me take a blood test because she wanted to stay healthy for Harry.

The people in a locked psychiatric unit are not the mentally ill people you see on TV ads, the All Blacks who have been to hell and back with depression and come out the other side. These are not the people who made the brave step to go to their GP and get an anti-depressant and a referral to a counsellor, and feel much better. I don't mean to diminish the suffering that people with common mental illnesses like anxiety and depression face; it is genuine, and profound. But people as unwell as the patients we cared for at Tiaho Mai are often left behind by campaigns to reduce the stigma of mental health, their illnesses too frightening to be easily relatable, and too unremitting to fit a hopeful narrative.

Schizophrenia is an illness that, without effective manage-ment, robs sufferers of duration and quality of life. Psychotic exacerbations are the most common reason that people with schizophrenia need to come into hospital, and these will usually respond to medication or, failing that, ECT. We call psychosis a 'positive symptom' of schizophrenia, not to say that it is a positive thing to happen, but because it adds something: a delusion, a hallucination or disorganised thinking. Negative symptoms of schizophrenia subtract something: facial expressions, motivation or the ability to enjoy life. Negative symptoms are much harder for us to treat, and over time make it harder for a person living with schizophrenia to live independently. Many of our patients lived in supported accommodation.

After the patient interviews were done for the day, it was time for our medical clinic. As the house officers on the team, Brittany and I looked after physical health while the psychiatrists and psychiatric registrars looked after mental health. A senior physician visited us most days to help us with medical management and answer any questions. We were brand new, and asked him for advice on nearly everything.

The theory was that every patient should have a medical history, basic physical examination, ECG and set of baseline blood tests within 24 hours of admission. This was important because psychiatric medications can cause physical side effects, blood test abnormalities and even occasionally heart rhythm disturbances. Perhaps unsurprisingly, these checks were often difficult to achieve in the first 24 hours — people with acute psychosis who have just been brought into a locked psychiatric unit against their will are generally not that excited about the prospect of letting a doctor attach electrodes to their chest or jab them with a needle.

Sometimes all we could safely do on the first day was watch them walking around the ward to confirm that they seemed to be alert, moving all four limbs, and not in pain. Once their mental health was stable enough, we would offer a medical consultation. Often, they declined, and we documented that we had asked, and offered again the next day.

To maximise our chances that patients would agree to be seen, we would usually wait to ask until people had finished cooking or arts and crafts or karaoke with the occupational therapists, so Brittany and I had a lot of downtime in our clinic room. We would sing old songs and gossip about our lives. We discovered that the brick phones we had been given as work phones could manually record a ringtone, and we set ours to a recording of Brittany singing 'ring, ring, ring'. Brittany wanted to see what her own ECG looked like, so we recorded one for her, and I had an overgrown cuticle so Brittany performed minor surgery on my nail. On Thursdays we would take our lunch early so that we could make it to the cafeteria before the cinnamon pinwheels ran out.

The nurses were our best asset in encouraging people to come to our clinic room. We would work as quickly as we could before patients lost interest or became frustrated. For people whose patience with us was particularly short, I would attach ECG leads while Brittany took a blood test. We would have them in and out in five minutes.

Psychiatric medications can work pretty fast, and once they had started to work, the patients were often very keen to see us. We were nice, friendly young doctors who could diagnose their aches and pains, order X-rays of old injuries they'd never had looked at, treat their rashes and earaches, and provide reassurance that the distressing body sensations that commonly accompany anxiety and depression were not actually going to kill them. We could refer them to the hospital dentists, who would perform tooth extractions and urgent fillings. The people we looked after were often living on very low incomes, and many of them had been living with toothache for a long time, so by the end of the rotation we were on a first-name basis with the hospital dentists.

We could also provide nicotine replacement. Most patients smoked, and because it was a no-smoking unit, they were desperate for a cigarette. We tried to keep them comfortable with patches, gum and lozenges, but every second conversation was still a plea to be allowed out for a smoke.

The most popular nicotine product was called the 'inhalator'. A small plastic tube roughly the size and shape of a cigarette, it had replaceable cartridges that provided nicotine, and was puffed on much like a cigarette. Inhalator was a misnomer — it wasn't a vape or an electronic cigarette, and the nicotine was released and absorbed in the mouth rather than actually being inhaled. But it gave people something to do with their hands, and even non-smokers on the ward would often ask for one. At one point, some of the young men started asking for new cartridges more often than we expected. The nurses investigated, and realised they had figured out how to light fires in their rooms using the power sockets in order to smoke the nicotine liquid in the cartridges. We were a little more judicious with the inhalators after that.

Patients were incredibly resourceful at sneaking cigarettes onto the ward. They would have their friends and family members bring smokes and lighters in food packages on visits. They would ask to be taken out to the shops to buy a phone or shoes, only to bring back cigarettes when they returned. Cigarette confiscations were a major source of conflict between patients and staff.

It must be an awful feeling to have your liberty, and your right to do something as simple as smoking a cigarette, taken away from you. I don't smoke, and I've never been sectioned, so no experience I have had can really compare. But I remember being in high school and getting in trouble for uniform violations (the wrong-coloured socks) or for drinking coffee in class. I remember how much I hated being in a place I didn't want to be, being told what to do, and being punished when I disobeyed.

A few of the patients ran away, but fewer than I would have expected from my memories of Hermione's time in hospital, in another city a decade ago. I think that was more because of the no-smoking policy and COVID than it was a reflection of our patients' enthusiasm for being in psychiatric care: the easiest way to escape had been during cigarette breaks or short walks outside, which were no longer allowed.

I did make a heroic attempt to chase one abscondee down as he strolled calmly straight past the security guard as if he was a visitor who was allowed to leave. I happened to be walking out to get a coffee at the same time, and I yelled out to the security guard. We both followed him, and the security guard radioed hospital security to help. They responded in a vehicle, and caught up with him about 500 metres down the road from the hospital, with the ward security guard hot on his heels, and a puffed Izzy trailing some way behind, ready to use my verbal de-escalation skills if they were needed. But he simply rolled his eyes and got into the security car to be brought back in.

You need a thick skin to work in psychiatry. The patients are unwell, disinhibited and often understandably furious at being locked up. I'm chubby, so the comments were mostly about my weight, with some occasional homophobia thrown in as well. One woman who needed weekly blood tests would scream, 'Ew, I'm not a fucking lesbian!' whenever I got near her with a needle (that famous sapphic mating ritual, phlebotomy). Kurt, petite in stature and with a staggering vocabulary, was insulted for being short and for being intelligent in roughly equal measure. Disappointingly, none of the patients made the obvious joke about a short shrink. For beautiful Brittany, it was mostly just sexual harassment. I would take the fat jokes over that any day.

Most of the assaults on us doctors were verbal. The nurses, who spent more time 'on the floor', were attacked physically, too. One patient committed an especially vicious assault on a nurse, completely out of the blue. Afterwards, he explained that he didn't want to be in hospital, and he figured if he assaulted someone he would get to go to jail instead.

Another patient, who was renowned for being impressively adept at destruction of property while unwell, shoved the nurse who was watching her so that she could run into the bathroom, lock the door, climb up on the toilet and tamper with the sprinklers to set them off. Chaos ensued and we had to evacuate. She apologised afterwards, sitting on carpet still wet from the sprinklers, and seemed to really mean it. I couldn't help but like her. She had a cheeky smile and a laugh that gurgled in her throat. Her mania was almost infectious, energising me even as I struggled to keep up with what she was saying.

The seclusion rooms were where a lot of new patients needed to go, if they posed an immediate danger of self-harm, or harm to staff or their fellow patients. Seclusion involved stark rooms, empty except for a mattress, adjacent to a lounge with a few big soft pieces of furniture, which were really mattresses in the shape of furniture, soft enough to be both soothing if sat upon and non-lethal if thrown. If the door between the rooms was open and the patient could move around freely, it was called 'retreat'. If the patient was locked in the room with the mattress, it was called 'seclusion'. Patients who came in screaming mad at being sectioned, or high on methamphetamine, often spent a few hours in retreat or seclusion to calm down before being taken to their room on the ward. Sedative medications could be given if appropriate, although the best option was to give antipsychotics, which would actually help the patient start to recover rather than just temporarily zonking them out.

A lot of our admissions came in after hours. The on-call

house officer would 'admit' these patients by looking up their medical history and writing an admission note, prescribing the psychiatric medications the registrar or consultant said were needed, charting nicotine replacement, and laying eyes on them to make sure they looked safe from a medical point of view. There were only five psychiatry house officers, so we had to do quite a lot of after-hours shifts to cover all the evenings and weekends. Most weeks we had two 'long days' (starting at 8.30 a.m. and finishing at 10 p.m.), and we worked every fifth weekend, two back-to-back long days in the middle of a twelve-day stretch.

Some long days were pretty relaxing, and one Sunday evening Brittany even managed to watch most of *Legally Blonde* in the office while drinking a cup of Milo. Others were chaotic. The psychiatry house officers also covered the stroke rehabilitation ward and the dementia ward after hours. Unlike a lot of our psychiatric patients who were relatively young and physically robust, the patients on those wards were frail and unwell, and we would often get called for the big three: fevers, falls and fluids.

One weekend I was called about the same patient falling over no fewer than five times. He had dementia, and never remembered to use his walking frame. Unless he was watched constantly, he would get up for a stroll and tumble over. It only took the nurse or healthcare assistant to turn their back for a second before he would be on the ground. Fortunately, he never seemed to hurt himself, but he also never remembered that he had fallen, and would be bewildered at why I was examining him from top to toe.

Dementia is a cruel illness. Some of the patients were what we called 'pleasantly confused' but others were agitated, frightened or aggressive. My only physical assault by a patient was an elderly man with dementia whom I was examining after a fall. I made the mistake of getting close enough that he could reach out and touch me, which he did, grabbing my breast hard and shouting 'I've got your boob!' at the top of his lungs. His favourite nurse scolded him for hurting the nice young doctor, and he let me go and asked for a cup of Milo.

I had a few other near misses, getting too close on more than one occasion to a patient prone to biting. Our lanyards were 'anti-choke' so that if a patient grabbed hold of them, they snapped open rather than tightening on our necks. Once or twice I was glad of that.

While after-hours calls from the stroke and dementia wards were usually for the same few problems, calls from the psychiatry wards could be for just about anything. We were called about earaches with the same sense of urgency other wards might reserve for chest pain. Occasionally, two patients would be caught having sex, and the house officer would have to review them, try to figure out if it had been consensual, and offer emergency contraception and STI screening. A colleague was once called after hours to provide first aid and fill out the occupational health form for two nurses because a patient had thrown a cup of piss in their faces, getting it in their eyes and mouths.

After three months as the psych house officer, watching what the nurses go through, I guess I could see how some of the people who were cruel to my friend Hermione might have become burnt out and stopped caring whether they were causing suffering. On one level, I have more empathy for them now. But I've also seen that the nurses I worked with at Tiaho Mai managed to work in those conditions and retain their humanity and their compassion. I have seen several nurses advocate for the patient who just assaulted them, and remind their colleagues that the person cannot help being unwell.

I thought that working in psychiatry would be awful, exposed to a behind-the-scenes look at how mistreatment of patients comes about. Certainly the resource constraints and the

Vital Signs

'bottom of the cliff' nature of acute mental-health care were frustrating and demoralising, and I met patients who I don't think would have been there if they'd had secure housing, a stable income and a supportive social network. But the staff I worked with were fierce protectors of their patients' dignity, and have given me hope for the future of mental-health care in this country. After trying so hard to get out of that job, I am very glad I didn't manage to do so.

The coolest thing in psychiatry is seeing people get better. When the psychiatrist gets the right combination of pills and they start to work, patients sometimes start returning to their former selves. This might be in a matter of days, or it might take months. For Hermione, it took years.

One young woman reminded me of Hermione a lot. She was on the ward for most of the time that Brittany and I worked at Tiaho Mai. She was virtually catatonic when we first met her, in a hospital gown with her hair dirty and matted. She didn't eat or speak. When she started to get a little better, she would have conversations with people we couldn't see or hear, and spent most of her free time shadow-boxing in the courtyard. The day she left Tiaho Mai, she was in a yellow sundress, her clean hair in a ponytail, laughing with another patient as they said goodbye.

The people with drug-induced psychosis got better quickly once the drugs were no longer in their system. We would send them home with advice to stay away from drugs in the future, because drugs didn't seem to agree with their brain chemistry. The people with schizophrenia took longer for their psychosis to improve, but it usually did eventually. We would discharge them back to the care of their usual community psych teams. Mania got better with the right dose of lithium. Day by day, the speech would slow and the train of thought would become easier to follow, until they were back at equilibrium.

After packing up my cubicle and moving on to work in the

main hospital, I would sometimes see old patients from Tiaho Mai around the wards, in hospital for health conditions or visiting family, free to live as they chose and smoke as much as they pleased. I smiled at them, and they smiled back.

CHAPTER 43

Graduation

WHEN I STARTED work, we hadn't yet had our med-school graduation. I took annual leave for the graduation ceremony, flew to Dunedin on Friday morning and picked up a rental car. It felt strange to be a visitor in the city I had lived in until two weeks previously, a city that had been my home for six years. My family were booked to fly in on Saturday morning. Both parents and a few of my siblings had arranged flights and accommodation, and I had managed to get extra tickets so they could all come to the ceremony. They had seen me graduate once before, with my Bachelor of Arts, but this was medicine. It was a big deal. My grandparents had decided it was too far for them to travel, so we had set them up with a link to the livestream.

I had time to catch up with a few friends before making my way to the airport to pick up Charlie from the afternoon flight. I got a coffee and a cinnamon scroll from Morning Magpie, and sat on the sunny lawn outside the railway station.

Vital Signs

By early afternoon, graduation had been cancelled. In a year of COVID cancellations, for once it wasn't the sneaky little virus that had decided to spoil our fun. Instead it was a security threat, and the university and police felt they couldn't guarantee everyone would be safe if the graduation ceremonies went ahead. My family decided they wouldn't come down after all. I was still doing the Oath Ceremony, and we had been looking forward to a weekend of visiting our old haunts, so Charlie kept her plans to fly down and join me.

Dunedin is one of my favourite places. I love the old buildings, the cool little cafes and the arty, alty people. I love the Otago Farmers' Market, the little theatre community, the poetry open mic nights and somehow running into the mayor, Aaron Hawkins, literally everywhere you go. I love vegan delis, summer gelato in the Octagon, and dinners at the waterfront in St Clair. I love the countless second-hand bookshops, and the very good University Bookshop, too. I love Port Chalmers, and I love the peninsula.

I had been living in Auckland for less than a month by that point, but flying back into Dunedin felt like coming home after many years abroad. It was familiar, and also strange. There were already new shops that I didn't recognise.

We were staying with my good friend Bryony and her two boys. I had lived with them for a few six-week stints in my nomadic sixth year of study, and it was from their house in Mornington that I had packed up my car in November bound for Auckland. Bryony set up the spare room for Charlie and me, and complimented me on my outfit and make-up as I got ready for the graduation ball.

I picked Charlie up from the airport and we made our way straight to the ball at the Otago Museum. A couple of hundred new doctors, along with partners and faculty members, were all gussied up and making short work of their allocated five drinks. I saw and hugged people I hadn't seen for three weeks, and people I hadn't seen for three years. I said 'Congratulations, Doctor!' about a hundred times. We shouted over the noise of the live band and danced to the usual crowd pleasers. Charlie and I gave a couple of our allocated drinks to two enterprising young law students who had managed to sneak into the med ball for the story, and were pretending they wanted to be surgeons when they grew up. I was exhausted from my first few weeks of work, so we slipped away to be in bed by midnight.

The next day was graduation day. Most of the university events had been cancelled: there would be no parade down George Street and no brunch in the Link. But we still had the two most important parts of medical graduation: the fancy certificate to one day put on our office walls, and the swearing of the Hippocratic Oath.

I remember reading an article once about a woman who 'married' her medical degree. She made wedding invitations, took engagement photos with her degree certificate, and threw a graduation party where she entered in a white dress and served a wedding cake. I think she was making a point about how our education and careers should be celebrated as much as (or more than) our romantic relationships, and I agree. In a way, standing up to take the Oath and commit my life to this profession really did feel like a wedding. Tears welled up in my eyes as I read the sacred words that bound me to so many other doctors — past, present and future.

Ka tāku hei Ika-ā-Whiro o te Kura Hauora o Te Whare Wānanga o Ōtākou
Ka eke atu te kounga o taku mahi whakaora tangata ki te tētahi taumata ikeike mōku me te ngākau tapatahi, te aroha pūmau, te kauanuanu anō hoki mō te oranga o te ira tangata,
Ka tukuna taku katoa kia tū hei pononga ki ngā tāngata katoa o te ao,

Vital Signs

Mā taku matatau me aku pūkenga ka ngana ki te whakapakari i te matatika o te tangata,

Me mātua tiaki ahau i taku oranga, i taku hauora kia taea ai e au te maimoa atu i te tangata ki tētahi paerewa tīkoke,

Ka whakautengia e au ngā kura huna kua munaia mai ki ahau,

Ka tū rangatira nei tēnei mahi ki a au, ko ōna uara, ko ōna mātāpono kia kake ai ko te oranga o te tangata tonu ki te akitu o whakahirahira.

Ka āta mātau au i aku taunahua me ngā pūkenga o tangata kē ki te whakatau māuiui, ki te ārai māuiui, ki te maimoa i te tangata,

Ka aro pū atu taku mahi kia ora pai ai rātou katoa ka noho ki raro i taku haumarutanga

A, ko te oranga tonutanga o te marea whānui hoki te kaupapa matua.

⌐

I undertake that as a graduate of Medicine at the University of Otago

I will practise the science and art of medicine to the best of my ability with moral integrity, compassion and respect for human dignity,

I will dedicate my life to the service of humanity,

I will use my knowledge and ability to further the realisation of human rights,

I will attend to my own health, well-being, and abilities in order to provide care of the highest standard,

I will respect the secrets which are confided in me,

I will honour the profession, its values and its principles in the ways that best serve the interests of patients,

I will recognise my own limitations and the special skills of others in the diagnosis, prevention and treatment of disease,
I will work for the good of all persons whose health may be placed in my care,
And for the public good.

Our graduation address was from Professor David Murdoch, the head of the Christchurch campus at the time, and who has since been made vice-chancellor of the whole university. He reflected on the many crises he had seen students and doctors respond to in his time in Christchurch: the earthquakes, floods, fires, the mosque shootings, and now a pandemic.

He told us about a World Health Organization meeting he had attended five years earlier in Geneva, in the wake of the Ebola outbreak in West Africa. The purpose of the meeting was to improve global readiness for future outbreaks of infectious disease. The group of global experts agreed on the need to be more prepared, and to help societies become stronger and more resilient. They hoped that the increased interest in public health due to Ebola could be harnessed to effect change. And yet, when the time came to respond to COVID-19, Professor Murdoch said he was not sure that we were any further ahead in our thinking and approach than five years earlier.

The recovery phase of the pandemic meant a similar period of thinking and planning would be underway here and across the globe, and he challenged us to make that work truly transformative.

'Quite frankly, graduates, I don't trust the generations ahead of you to do this alone. We don't have a great track record, and there is a real danger that we will return to business as usual. So, we need your help. We need you to be the agents of change.'

Hearing that, I felt equal parts inspired and sad. For most of my life I have been someone who questions the status quo. It is a polarising quality: some leaders find it refreshing, while others seem to find it threatening, and it would be fair to say that I have not entirely perfected the art of diplomacy (the phrase 'bull in a china shop' comes to mind). I have refined my approach slightly since the days of protesting against my school's uniform policy by spray-painting my shoes, but I am still a fairly blunt instrument of change.

With six years of study in medicine under my belt, I had already seen how easy it was for all of us idealistic students to come to accept that some things we at first found hard to swallow were 'just the way things are'. The culture shock of starting the fourth year of medical school had left me exhausted and disillusioned, but that had given way to a belief that I have to survive the health system as it is now if I want to change it. I had already seen how vulnerable young doctors are to the opinions of their seniors. Medicine is political, and junior doctors are always just one mediocre reference away from missing out on the competitive surgical training programme or the sought-after fellowship position.

Listening to Prof Murdoch's challenge I wondered whether, if push comes to shove, I have it in me to fight injustice if the fight is career-limiting, or isolates me from my peers. I wondered if the desire to succeed, and the desire to be liked, mean that one day I will be the one shrugging as people junior to me say that the system isn't working, and the one telling them it's just how things are.

In a medical humanities group I used to go to, I met a senior doctor who was part of the class of medical students in Wellington who refused to perform vaginal examinations on anaesthetised patients without consent, leading to the practice changing. I'm sure she won't mind me saying that she's not a young doctor now, and this wasn't especially recent, but she is also still within her working life, which makes it altogether too recent for me.

The story made me shudder because I had been previously unaware that this practice was common in New Zealand within living memory, but it also gave me hope. The most junior members of the medical profession had managed to lead a fundamental change through passive resistance. There would have been immense social pressure on them to just go with the flow and carry out the examination. Throughout my training there has been an expectation that medical students will be seen and not heard, will be minimally annoying, and will seize the opportunities presented to them (and I am sure this would have been seen as an opportunity).

By today's ethical standards, I don't think I have participated in any violations of patient rights quite so egregious as that one, but I have certainly made the decision not to rock the boat in the interests of self-preservation. I have stayed silent while others have made discriminatory jokes, even when the jokes made me flinch. I have chosen to fight senior doctors' unkind words to patients or colleagues by coming back to check on the person later, rather than by raising the issue with the senior doctor concerned. Maybe that is how it begins, how you start to be someone who preserves the status quo more than you challenge it.

After the Oath ceremony and Professor Murdoch's speech, we had some lunch and then went to the university campus to collect my degree certificate. I got a photo with Vice-Chancellor Harlene Haynes, who had received dozens of emails about injustice from me during my six years as a student. We took photos in front of the clocktower where I had pasted posters in protest at the university's censorship of the student magazine. We walked along the pavers where I had joined a rally in support of the humanities when the university had slashed their funding. I made myself a silent promise not to stop being an activist now that my student days were finally behind me.

Vital Signs

We went out for dinner with some close friends, and Charlie gave me the most beautiful bunch of flowers. In the morning, we had brunch and made our way to the airport. I held my precious piece of paper in my lap on the flight, scared it would bend in my carry-on. My eyes prickled as the plane wheels left Dunedin tarmac. It wasn't home anymore.

The next morning I drove to Middlemore Hospital, crossed the footbridge, waited at the traffic crossing, showed the security guard my staff ID. *Dr Isabelle Lomax-Sawyers, House Officer*. It was my third week of work, but the first time the title didn't make me feel like an imposter. I was a graduate of Otago Medical School. I had dedicated my life to the service of humanity. I was a doctor.

CHAPTER 5

Rhythms

BOTH BRITTANY AND I moved on to orthopaedic surgery after we finished at Tiaho Mai, and I joined a team with Sam and Gaby. It was in orthopaedics that I really learned how to be a house officer.

We were the Wednesday team, meaning that our team saw new patients and ran the acute operating theatre on Wednesdays. Two of our consultants were spinal surgeons, while the others specialised in foot and ankle surgery. I had never done an orthopaedic run in medical school, so I knew the specialty by reputation alone.

If clinical medicine was an American high-school movie, the two biggest cliques would be those working in medicine and those working in surgery. Surgeons have a reputation as the popular kids, the Jocks (orthopaedic surgeons), and the Plastics (self-explanatory). They live in nice houses, wear nice clothes and drive nice cars, which they buy with the money they earn working in nice clinics and nice operating theatres in the private system a couple of days a week. The occasional surgeon works only in the public system on principle; this is oft-remarked upon among juniors in hushed, adoring tones.

Medical specialties are for the nerds. These are the kids in chess club and debate club, the science fair winners, the band geeks. They are very brainy, and use their knowledge of how bodies and medications work to treat patients. There is a nerd hierarchy, with the prestigious procedural specialties like cardiology and the terribly complicated specialties like renal medicine at the top, the depressing but noble specialties like oncology and haematology somewhere in the middle, and general medicine, the busy service that looks after the patients without a home anywhere else, right at the bottom.

The arty kids, the theatre kids, the goths and the burnouts probably end up in general practice or psychiatry. The class clowns end up in ED and put their ADHD to good use. The do-gooders who like themselves end up in paediatrics, and the do-gooders who hate themselves (or at least hate sleep) end up in obstetrics and gynaecology.

I'm not from a medical family, and didn't really know any doctors socially. The only doctors I had met before medical school were ED doctors and GPs who had treated me on the odd occasion when I had been injured or ill. And so until perhaps my fourth year, the details of the medical hierarchy and the different specialties were a mystery to me.

I'm not alone in this. Hospital patients are frequently confused by who is in charge, and what their job title is. Age can provide a clue, but only a clue — as a house officer I am the most junior member of the team, but as a mature student I am not always the youngest. Add in stereotyping about gender and ethnicity and it's not uncommon for patients to ask their questions of the white male medical student instead of the Māori female consultant.

At the head of every medical team is a consultant, or a group of consultants. In medicine, the term 'consultant' doesn't mean they work for a private firm and charge megabucks. It's just the job title for a fully qualified doctor who is registered as a specialist in their field and has a whole bunch of letters after their name, also called a 'senior medical officer' or SMO. On American television shows this person is the 'Attending' and they are 'board certified'. In Australia and New Zealand, this certification is through one of the medical 'colleges'. The consultant is the doctor ultimately responsible for the care a patient receives.

The next step down from a consultant is the registrar. They are a doctor training in that area of specialty, but not yet fully qualified. They are the person responsible for overseeing the day-to-day care of patients. They have enough experience to manage simple problems without much input from the consultant, and they provide leadership to the more junior members of the team.

The term 'registrar' means different things in different countries. In New Zealand, registrar can mean anything from a third-year doctor just 'stepping up', all the way to perhaps a doctor with ten or fifteen years' experience about to take their final subspecialty exams. In the UK, 'senior house officer' seems to be used for the more junior part of that training journey.

In some fields, especially surgery, the distinction is made between a 'training registrar' who already has a place in the coveted surgical training programme (and is therefore more senior), and a 'non-training registrar' who is more junior and still trying to impress and gain a spot on the programme. In all the hospitals I've worked in, surgical teams have a senior registrar who is a trainee, and a junior registrar who isn't. Our orthopaedic team had one senior registrar and two junior regs. The senior registrar spends most of their time operating, or seeing patients in clinic. The junior registrar spends some time in theatre learning operations, some time in clinics, and admits new patients in ED. The juniors are usually available during the day to answer questions from the house officers, and to help troubleshoot issues that arise with patients on the wards.

The next step down is me, the house officer. The house officer is the most junior doctor on the team, usually in her first or second year of work, although third-year doctors who haven't settled on a specialty or are waiting for a job to come up often keep working as an 'HO'. The house officer is responsible for the tasks that need to be done to take care of our team's patients. We take notes on ward rounds, order blood tests and scans and chase the results, insert IV lines and catheters, prepare admission and discharge paperwork, chart medications and are usually the first medical eyes to review any new symptoms that the patients report to the nurses. In some hospitals, big surgical teams will have two, or even three, house officers. Medical teams usually just have one.

Some countries make a distinction between the first and second year of being a doctor, with the first year called an internship. In Australia, first-year doctors are called interns, while doctors in their second year or later who don't yet have a registrar job are called residents. In New Zealand, the medical council technically refers to first- *and* second-year doctors as interns, but the term is rarely used at work.

The next member of the medical team is a trainee intern, or final-year medical student. They have done most of the learning about basic medicine they need to step up to being a doctor, and are now learning the job of the house officer. They do many of the same tasks as a house officer, but under close supervision. They don't have prescribing rights, so they practise charting medications and then get the house officers to sign off.

The more junior medical students on the team are there to learn about the specialty, and they mostly follow the registrars and consultants. On the ward round, it is their responsibility to pull the curtain closed at each patient bedspace, and to find the notes. They provide light banter and, on the last day of their rotation, baking.

Every weekday, some combination of the doctors and students in the medical team do a ward round to see all the patients under their care. I say ward round, although perhaps it should be *wards* round. In all but the smallest or most organised hospitals, a team will be looking after patients on multiple wards, potentially in multiple buildings. Half of the ward round is taken up by walking. At Middlemore, we called this a 'safari ward round'. The registrar typically leads the safari (the consultant is far too busy thinking important thoughts to figure out where the round needs to go next).

The consultants will quietly grumble when the registrars leading a ward round get the order wrong and have to double back, and I heard of one consultant surgeon at another hospital who, if his juniors accidentally missed a ward and had to turn back, would make the whole team walk to the bottom of the stairs, all the way up to the top floor and then back down as punishment.

There are two basic types of ward round in any hospital. The first is a surgical ward round. The surgical ward round starts at the crack of dawn so that the registrars can get to clinic and the consultants can get to theatre. At Middlemore, surgical house officers come in early to 'prep the list' by writing down blood results the consultant might ask for, and checking the patient's overnight vital signs. A prepped list might also include how many days since the operation, a reminder of which bug we are treating (based on the bacteria found in the patient's blood, in tissue samples or on swabs), what antibiotic we are using and for how long, and what measures are being used to prevent blood clots while the patient is laid up in bed. This is usually Clexane, an anti-clotting medicine injected into the tummy, and tight compression stockings called TEDs. Sam, Gaby and I were meticulous in prepping our list, and it was detailed and neat.

The orthopaedic surgery ward round starts at 6.45. All the patients are asleep, the night nurses are trying to use the patient charts to write their shift notes before handover, and none of the blood tests for the day are back yet. While the house officer has been preparing the list, the registrar has been marching around the ward with a big pair of shears, going into the rooms of selected patients and cutting down bandages painstakingly wrapped by the nurses.

The team of doctors and students then marches up and down the ward at speeds rivalling a pack of Olympic power-walkers. The house officer is unofficially responsible for smiling and greeting any receptionists, nurses, social workers and physios whom the rest of the team has ignored while striding past. The medical students are unofficially responsible for carrying the equipment needed on an orthopaedic round: a tendon hammer, sterile drapes to temporarily cover any wounds that the team has un-bandaged, and a spare pair of plaster shears.

Seeing each patient takes about two minutes. There is a brief 'How are you?' and then a quick look at the limb of interest. Tales are whispered in junior doctor lounges of orthopaedic ward rounds where the consultant has pronounced that a limb looks good without noticing that the patient who owns the limb has died. I *think* that is just urban legend.

The format most commonly used for clinical notes in New Zealand is 'SOAP' — subjective, objective, assessment (most commonly rephrased as 'impression' in practice) and plan.

Date
CWR (consultant ward round) Surname [or]
RWR (registrar ward round) Surname
Time

Subjective   *What has been discussed with the patient.
Might include how they are feeling, whether
they have passed urine and opened their
bowels, if they are sleeping well. Will also
include whether we have broken bad news or
discussed the possible complications of
a procedure.*

Objective   *Vital signs, examination findings, relevant
blood results. (Often headed up O/E —
on examination).*

Impression   *The diagnosis, or a comment about how the
patient is recovering, or both.*

Plan   *Some combination of instructions to the
nurses and a list of things the doctors
intend to do for the patient. On the fastest
of ward rounds, the plan might just be
'cont' (continue).*

In Orthopaedics, by the time the house officer has found the file, opened it to the right page, and written the date, time, and the consultant or registrar's name, it's time to move on to the next patient. Fortunately, these short ward-round consultations can be communicated in only a few letters.

Vital Signs

L) ankle trimalleolar #.
N afeb, NVI
NBM for OT, BMC
NWB

Orthopaedic ward round glossary

*fracture*

N afeb   *vital signs are within normal limits, and the patient hasn't had a fever*

NVI   *neurovascularly intact. The nerves and blood vessels of the broken limb don't appear to be damaged.*

E+D   *the patient is free to eat and drink*

NBM for OT   *please keep this patient nil by mouth, for operating theatre — we will potentially do their operation today*

BMC   *the patient needs to be booked for theatre, taken through a consent form by one of the junior doctors, and have a mark on the affected limb in a special medical Sharpie, so that we don't chop off the wrong leg while they are asleep*

NWB   *please keep this patient non-weight-bearing on the affected limb or digit*

WBAT   *the patient can weight-bear as tolerated*

Cont   *continue intravenous antibiotics*
IVAbx

POAbx   *oral antibiotics*

ID   *the house officer will call our esteemed
                colleagues in infectious diseases medicine
                for advice on this patient's antibiotics*

MDT   *kindly requesting input from our esteemed
                colleagues in physio and occupational
                therapy, with many thanks*

D/c   *discharge*

Sam, Gaby and I had our ward rounds down to a fine art. Two of us would push ahead and prepare the notes for the upcoming patients, while one of us stayed behind to listen to the ward round. Most of our notes would already be written by the time the surgeons reached the bedside.

A registrar round on 'old patients' is usually finished by 7.30 a.m. A consultant round after the weekend might last a little longer, perhaps until 8.30. On days when the team is 'post-acute' (meaning that the previous day you were admitting new patients), the power-walking might last until 10 a.m. This is usually followed by a team coffee bought by the most senior member of the team. Most days, the orthopaedic surgeons and their juniors are at coffee before General Medicine (Gen Med) has even finished morning handover.

People come to the orthopaedic ward with two basic problems: something is broken, or something is infected. I am sure the orthopaedic surgeons could list a dozen ways in which this is an over-simplification, but they are busy at the golf course.

Vital Signs

If something is broken, it needs to be fixed. Fortunately, human bodies are miraculous and can often fix themselves, making new bone tissue to repair breaks. A blood clot forms, and the chemicals released through inflammation act as a fire siren, telling the cells that will be needed for healing to show up like a swarm of nanobot firefighters. Cells called fibroblasts spit out simple scar tissue. Bone cells called osteoblasts spit out bone material. As long as the broken ends are held still enough, the bone heals.

A few things can screw up this healing process. Some of them are what we would call 'patient factors': smoking, high blood sugar, poor circulation and poor nutrition. But there are some things that orthopaedic treatment can address directly: keeping a bone still enough to heal, and treating or preventing infection.

To keep the ends of a bone still, you can either wrap it in a cast from outside, or do some carpentry to join it back together. The commonest surgical method of fixing a fracture is called open reduction and internal fixation (ORIF). When we are talking about fractures, 'reduction' just means putting the displaced pieces of bone back where they belong, and 'fixation' means making sure they stay there. So an open reduction means cutting the soft tissues open and getting the bones back in a good position, and internal fixation means holding the bone ends into place with plates, screws, nails, wires and other metalware that stays inside the body.

Another method of fixing a fracture is with pins and wires inserted through the skin, and held by a scaffolding frame that sits outside the body. We call this external fixation or ex-fix. The advantage of this is that it can be used in some situations where internal fixation can't, or can be used to quickly and temporarily hold the bones in place when more life-threatening injuries are being taken care of (such as in a major trauma). The major disadvantage that I can see is that it looks like a medieval torture device. When my granny was in a car accident, the scariest thing about seeing her in the hospital was the metal contraption drilled into her leg.

Finally, if a joint is absolutely buggered, it might need a replacement. This is often the case when an elderly person comes in with a broken hip, but shoulders and knees can be replaced too.

The other orthopaedic problem, infection, can be in the skin (cellulitis), a joint (septic arthritis) or the bone (osteomyelitis). There are also abscesses — pockets of pus which have collected in the tissues. All these types of infections can be pretty bad. Perhaps the worst infection of all is necrotising fasciitis, known colloquially as 'flesh-eating disease'. I haven't seen it yet, and I'm grateful.

There are two ways to get rid of the bacteria that cause an infection. One is to kill them with antibiotics. Different antibiotics kill different bugs, and when you are first treating an infection you don't know what bug you're dealing with, so you use something pretty broad. It's your best guess as to which antibiotics should work on the types of bacteria that usually cause infections in that part of the body. We call that empiric treatment.

Before starting the broad-spectrum antibiotic, we try to get a sample of the bacteria we are dealing with to send to the lab. We take a blood sample in case the bacteria is in the blood. We take swabs of any pus discharging from the wound. If the person needs an operation, we save a sample of any dead tissue we removed. Then, while the broad antibiotic is working on killing the bacteria, our lab staff can get to work on telling us exactly which bug we're dealing with, and which antibiotics will kill it.

Why go to so much trouble, when we have a broad-spectrum antibiotic that can treat the infection? Well, certain antibiotics only kill certain bacteria until they don't. Every time we expose bacteria to an antibiotic, we kill the bacteria that *are* susceptible to that antibiotic, and encourage the few bacteria that are starting to develop resistance to live and breed. It's a zombie apocalypse where with every spray of bullets at a pack of zombies, most of them die but a few of them get stronger.

By switching to the narrowest antibiotic that will kill only the actual bug we're dealing with, we are saving the broad-spectrum antibiotics for when we really need them.

(If the infectious diseases registrar from my first year reads this, he will be shocked to discover that I do actually know the basic principles of antibiotic treatment. Despite this, as soon as I have a patient I am worried about, even when we know the bacteria we are treating and what antibiotics it is sensitive to, I am on the phone asking if we can have an antibiotic of last resort as a little treat. We need the infectious diseases doctors to save us from ourselves.)

The second way to remove bacteria that are causing an infection is literally to remove them. Drain the big collection of pus. Remove the metalware that is colonised by bacteria. Cut away the infected tissue. In extreme cases, amputate the infected limb. We call this source control. Remove the source of infection, and the patient gets better. Leave the source of infection intact, and antibiotics alone might not be enough to treat it.

Orthopaedics is satisfying because (often) there is a problem and a solution. The bone is broken, we operate, the bone heals straight. There is a knee joint full of pus, we drain it, the patient feels better. The patient comes to us with a broken hip, we fix it, and they get to live a little longer. For all the fun I like to poke at orthopaedic surgeons, I am truly in awe of the things they can do to give patients quantity and quality of life.

If an orthopaedic ward round is Olympic power-walking, a medical ward round is aqua jogging: working very hard to move forwards very slowly.

On a medical ward round, the team will huddle around a computer with the files for a few of the patients on the list. The most senior people will be sitting down and the juniors stand behind them.

Lengthy preparation takes place before we go in to see the patient. A good medical ward-round note starts with a problem list. This is a list of things the patient is currently being treated for, and a brief summary of the treatment. It might go something like this:

> *76F*
> *New AF, commenced diltiazem. CHADSVASc = 5,*
> *HASBLED = 1. Commenced rivaroxaban.*
> *Decompensated HF 2' to 1), on IV frusemide*
> *HAP on IV cef*
> *T2DM on Galvumet*

What does this mean? A 76-year-old woman who was admitted with atrial fibrillation has been started on medicine to prevent her heart from going too fast. A clinical scoring tool for people with AF indicates that she is at relatively high risk of a stroke, and a tool for checking her risk of bleeding on blood thinners shows that the benefits of blood thinners should outweigh the risk. A blood thinner has been started. She's also had some heart failure because of her heart going too fast, and is on a diuretic to offload extra fluid. While in hospital she has acquired pneumonia and is on IV antibiotics for that. She's also type II diabetic, and is on oral medication to control her blood sugar.

The registrar or consultant will personally look through the blood test results and vital signs, check the bowel chart to see if the patient is constipated, and review what medications are prescribed.

When it's finally time to see the first patient, they'll sit down at the bedside for a long chat, while the poor house officer stands in the background scribbling notes into the ring binder, and the medical students crowd awkwardly behind. Then they'll examine whether the patient has too much fluid on board or not enough, listen to the heart and lungs, and do any more specialised examination that might be needed depending on the patient's diagnosis. The most helpful bosses and registrars will tell the house officer the examination findings as they go. The less helpful will leave us to guess.

Finally, they'll explain to the patient what they think is wrong, and what they plan to do about it. One of my favourite bosses in medical school was a brilliant physician called Dr Chatterjee. He used the same script for this part of every consultation, and I heard it so many times that even now, four years later, I can recite it word for word. 'Thank you for answering my questions, sorry for the poking and the prodding. Here's what we'll do.'

Sometimes of their own accord, and sometimes with a nudge from the house officer, the consultant dictates their impression. *Decompensated heart failure — improving*. Then they'll list any extra parts of the plan that weren't mentioned when they explained it to the patient. Dr Chatterjee would even dictate bullet points and sub bullet points, including instructions for precisely what to do if there were problems after hours.

A short medical ward round is finished by lunchtime. The longest I have seen was still going at 9 p.m. At that point, the last patient to see would surely be the house officer, presenting with papercuts, exhaustion and serious questions about their chosen career.

The longest ward rounds are usually on days when there are new patients on the list, admitted the night before. Every department has a system for deciding who will take care of new patients. Usually, each team within the department will be assigned a certain day of the week when all patients referred to the specialty by GPs or ED doctors come in under their care. A day when your team is admitting patients is your 'acute day'.

The day after an acute day is a 'post-acute' day, when your team has brand-new patients who will all need to be seen by a consultant on the 'post-acute ward round'. Post-acute days are the busiest days of the week.

Someone from the team of doctors will see every patient on their list every weekday. At least a few times a week this will be the consultant, with the rest of the team in tow. On days when the consultant isn't doing a ward round, the registrar will see the patients, and discuss them with the consultant afterwards. On some services, the ward round will sometimes be done by the house officer.

Different departments and different hospitals seem to approach the weekends differently. Some departments round on every patient on both weekend days. Other departments see every patient on a Saturday ward round, but on Sundays only see patients who are new, or patients who are very sick. In some big and busy departments, only new patients and patients who have been 'put up for review' on a weekend handover list get seen by doctors over the weekend.

The lighter workload without weekend ward rounds means that we can maintain a basic Monday to Friday working week, and then share out the after-hours duties equally. Every house officer and registrar is rostered to stay at work for one or two long days every week, covering any urgent tasks that need to be done from 4 p.m. until handover around 10 p.m. Consultants are rostered to be on call (usually for a full 24 hours), and will stay after hours if things are busy, and come back in if the registrar asks them to. Every few weeks we work the weekend, and every month or two we work a set of nights. Our salary for a rotation depends on how many long days and weekends are on the roster, as well as how many unrostered hours we are expected to work.

Orthopaedics was among the better-paid rotations, as we worked an average of 60–65 hours per week, with higher pay

Vital Signs

making up for the lack of a social life. It meant we could easily afford the several coffees we bought every day to counteract the sleep deprivation. The early starts and short winter days meant we barely saw the sun for three months.

CHAPTER 6:

Nurses

HEALTHCARE RELIES ON teamwork. If you're ever in hospital, the team who look after you will include between five and ten people all with different job titles. You'll probably see a phlebotomist, who will collect a blood sample from you to help with diagnosis. You might need a scan, to which you'll be wheeled by an orderly, and which will be taken by a radiographer. While you're on the ward, you might see a physiotherapist. If you're injured, they will check that you can get around safely, and teach you to use crutches or a walking frame if you need it. If you have a chest infection, or have just had an operation, they might give you some breathing exercises.

You might see an occupational therapist, who will figure out what equipment can help you to care for yourself safely at home. You might need to see a social worker, who can help you to organise personal carers or meals on wheels, or who can help you to get a place in a rest home. If you're having a hard time with a new diagnosis, you might be seen by a health

Vital Signs

psychologist. You might be washed or taken to the toilet by a healthcare assistant. A cleaner will empty the rubbish and clean your room. Kitchen staff will take your meal order every day, and deliver your food to the ward. A receptionist will help your family and friends find you when they visit. Once or twice a day, you'll see your doctors. But there is nobody you'll see more of than your nurse.

A nurse will check your vital signs at the beginning of the shift, and at least every four hours after that, plotting it all on a graph. They'll bring you medications whenever they're due, and call the doctor on your behalf if they think there are medications you need that aren't prescribed. They'll care for your IV luers (valves) to prevent infection. They'll answer the call bell when you ring it, fill your water jug, bring you a cup of tea when you ask. They'll measure exactly how much water you've had to drink, and how much urine is coming out in your catheter. They'll put you on the bedpan and clean you up when you're done. If you have a scan or procedure planned for the day, they'll call to make sure it is going ahead, and to find out what time.

If you can't move on your own, your nurse will turn you to prevent pressure sores. They'll answer the phone when your family calls, and explain what is wrong with you and how you are getting on. When you're frustrated or tired or sore, you'll complain to a nurse, and they'll hopefully show you sympathy. When the doctors haven't done something we said we'd do, it's a nurse who will call to remind us, and risk getting told off. When doctors want to make sure that something happens for our patient that day, the person we talk to is the nurse.

Every member of the healthcare team is essential, but perhaps nobody more so than the nurses. There are never enough nurses. Every place I have worked has been chronically short-staffed, scrambling to plug gaps left by sick leave and resignations, asking nurses to work double shifts for sixteen hours or more.

It's easy to see why nursing teams are short-staffed: the pay comes nowhere close to rewarding the level of skill, dedication and care required to do a good job, or even an okay job. And honestly, some of the patients are arseholes. You'd be hard pressed to find a nurse who hasn't been sworn at, spat at or groped in the line of duty. Then there are the patients who get delirium while unwell, and who through no fault of their own turn from sweet grandmas to vicious martial artists intent on using their still-attached catheter bag as a weapon.

As if all of that wasn't enough, nurses also have to deal with nonsense from junior doctors like me who have been working for all of five minutes. The relationship between nurses and doctors is one of the closest working relationships in the hospital, and also one of the most fraught. I don't think we are very good at understanding the challenges of one another's jobs.

Nurses contribute majorly to our workload. They make most of the hundreds of phone calls we receive every week. They put up all the tasks on our Task Manager. During the day, they call to remind us to do jobs that are already on our impossibly long to-do list. After hours, they call us to review patients. Sometimes this is because the patients need to be reviewed, and other times it is to get the patient off the nurse's back.

> *Patient is complaining of cough — please review (patient in hospital with pneumonia).*

> *Patient is feeling upset because their scan was postponed and needs a review.*

> *Patient is still waiting for discharge papers (call received while the doctor is on hour six of the post-acute ward round, is keenly aware of the jobs piling up but can't make the round go any faster, and hasn't had lunch).*

Vital Signs

Patient is complaining about the quality of the bed linen (prefers silk pillowcase) — please review.

But we house officers contribute majorly to the nursing workload too. If we are worried about a patient, we might ask their nurse to do vital-signs recordings more frequently, do 'neuro obs' to monitor for head injury, record a strict fluid balance, and monitor urine output every two hours or even hourly. Sometimes this is actually necessary, and the nurses are happy to do it. Other times it is requested because the house officer doesn't really understand what they are asking of the nurse, and they will roll their eyes at us. We put patients on IV antibiotics that are time-consuming to draw up and administer, or on insulin infusions that require the nurse to constantly monitor blood sugar and adjust the rate of insulin. If patients are very sick, the level of care we will ask their nurse to give is practically impossible while also juggling the tasks needed for other patients. It is through the dedication of the whole nursing team that, most of the time, our requests are met.

Outside of an ICU setting, most nurses are looking after between three and seven patients, which means taking a blood pressure, heart rate, oxygen level, respiratory rate and temperature every four hours at minimum, managing all IV infusions and regular medications, answering the near-constant call bells, giving 'PRN' (pro re nata, which means 'as needed') medications like pain relief, anti-nausea medicine and laxatives when the patients request them, answering phone calls from family members hoping for an update, and giving emotional support to patients who are frightened, sore and miserable. It's a hard, exhausting job, so much so that for most nurses, full-time work 'on the floor' is 32 hours a week.

Nurses have saved my arse on more than one occasion. They follow up on jobs that I have genuinely forgotten to do. They picked up the time I inadvertently prescribed something a patient was allergic to. They notice when patients aren't doing too well, even if it is just the 'I can't put my finger on it, but something's not right' spidey sense that is hard to justify but perilous to ignore.

The best ones call me with a solution as well as a problem. One surgical nurse, Chelsea, was especially good at this. She was beloved by house officers because she put in her own IV lines, had a wicked sense of humour, and didn't take bullshit from anyone. With several years' experience in surgical nursing, she definitely knew more than I did about a lot of the work we did together, and we both knew it.

'Hey, Iz, I've got a patient whose vascular surgery wound is oozing quite a lot. Often when this happens, the team withhold the Clexane. Thoughts on me doing that?'

If a nurse like Chelsea calls me, worried enough to ask me to come and see a patient, I know that I need to drop everything and do that straight away. Getting to know the nurses on the different wards is one of the nicest things about rotating through the hospital, and one of the saddest things about the end of each run.

CHAPTER 7:

Darkness

THE ALARM GOES off at 5.30 a.m. I don't hit snooze; it's day nine of a ten-day stretch, and I'm too tired to bargain with myself for five more minutes in my warm bed. I roll out of Charlie's arms and put a pillow in my place. She stirs for a moment, then hugs it and rolls over. It's pitch black and I turn on my phone torch so I can see what I'm doing. I have learned the hard way that a little bit of light is less disruptive to Charlie's sleep than the noise of me trying to get ready in total darkness. I grab some clean undies from the drawer, sending a silent prayer of thanks to the universe for Charlie, who has done my laundry and saved me from a possible underwear crisis. I throw on trackpants, a hoodie and my work sneakers. I drop my car keys on the floor, and Charlie groans. I whisper an apology, give her a kiss and creep out the door.

It's dark outside. I get into my little Yaris and put in an online order for my morning coffee from the only place that's open that early: the petrol station down the road. It's a hazelnut latte day, a morning when I'm so tired that the only thing that might wake me up enough for ward rounds is a sugary burst of hazelnut syrup. I choose a new audiobook to borrow on the library's app, which I'll listen to over a couple of weeks on the twenty-minute drive to and from work. *Uglies*, by Scott Westerfeld, catches my eye. It was a favourite as a teenager, and I haven't read it in years. I download it and press play.

My coffee is ready when I arrive, and I give the barista a tired smile. The only other people at the petrol station this early are construction workers, tradies and truck drivers. I give a friendly nod to a couple of lads in hi vis, and take my precious milky cargo back to the car. I grab my breakfast out of the glovebox: a hazelnut muesli bar, the closest thing to a proper breakfast that I can stomach at 5.30 a.m. I take one of the antihistamines that I keep in the car so I won't forget them, washing it down with a swig of coffee. Mm, hazelnutty. I take a bite of my muesli bar and start the car.

My flat is about a one-minute drive from the on-ramp to the Southern Motorway, the fastest way to Middlemore. At that time of day there is barely anyone on the road. I drink my coffee and chomp my muesli bar as the audiobook introduces the protagonist, Tally Youngblood.

The drive to work takes me twenty minutes at that time of day. When I arrive at the Middlemore staff car park I fumble in the car door pocket for my parking card. The balance flashes: $2.44. I'm pretty sure it's the day my weekly pass renews, and I'll need to top up before leaving work. This early, I can usually get a ground-floor park. I spot one, and pull in. I throw back the last few glugs of coffee and chuck the empty cup in the coffee-cup graveyard on the passenger side's floor. I need to clean my car.

I climb the footbridge over the train line, then walk down on the hospital side. There are no cars around, and I ignore the passenger signals and cross the road to the main entrance. I greet the night security guard, a Pasifika woman in her sixties who smiles at me as I show my card to her like I do every morning. Other than sleeping Charlie and the folk at the petrol station, she is the first person I see every day. On long days, I see her when I leave the hospital at the start of her shift, and when I arrive back in the morning at the start of mine.

I trudge down the Rainbow Corridor, take the lift to the theatre changing rooms, and get into scrubs. I love scrubs. I love the baggy drawstring trousers too long for my stubby legs, and the deep trouser pockets perfect for sinking your hands into. I love the smock-like scrub tops with their huge patch pockets, which can hold the three phones I have to carry on night shifts, a huge handful of spare pens, my folded-up patient list and even a snack. I love the different colours, which can tell people in the know what kind of doctor you are.

In Dunedin, students wore navy blue 'visitor' scrubs to theatre. The staff wore teal scrubs, and God help the medical student who was caught by the theatre nurses inadvertently wearing the staff ones. The only problem was that in the Emergency Department the consultants wore navy, and the ED nurses would give you sideways glances if you wore your navy scrubs when admitting patients in ED on surgical long days. The ED junior doctors wore a light powder blue, which was also worn by the obstetrics and gynaecology doctors and midwives. The ICU doctors wore whichever scrubs they felt like.

At Middlemore, the theatre scrubs are navy. ED doctors wear dark green scrubs with 'doctor' embroidered on them. Some of the medical doctors working with COVID patients wear powder blue, and some wear theatre blue.

Before COVID, it was only really the surgical and ED doctors who wore scrubs. The medical doctors usually wore smart casual 'clinical clothes'. During the Delta outbreak, I happily embraced the opportunity to wear what I call 'doctor pyjamas' every day in the name of hygiene. I can wear my activewear to work, get changed into my scrubs for the day, work my shift, get changed back into activewear, and put my scrubs in a laundry bag for someone else to wash. My closet is full of cute dresses and fun tops that are now only seen on my days off. I hope I can wear scrubs forever, regardless of what specialty I end up choosing.

Once I have changed, I take another lift to the top floor, to the orthopaedic wards, and dump my bag in the doctors' area, the 'fishbowl' as we fondly know it.

Gaby, Sam and I are on a busy team, and one of our trio is usually first to arrive; today it's me. The night house officer must be on another ward, or helping the registrar in ED, and is nowhere to be seen. I make myself an instant coffee in the nurses' break room, and get myself settled at a computer. I log in, open the programme we print our patient lists from, and tick my four consultants' names to generate the list of patients under their care. Then I log into our clinical portal and look up blood tests and vital signs so I can annotate the list.

Gaby arrives a few minutes later, a black crew sweatshirt over her scrubs, and deftly applied eye make-up almost disguising her tired eyes. She'd been on long day the night before, and factoring in travel time this means she has had roughly seven hours at home between yesterday's shift and today's. I'm already prepping the list, so she starts working on a discharge summary for a patient who should be transferred back to her rest home that day. The night house officer arrives back and greets us. She's had a busy night, with several 777s and an unexpected death. She starts working on printing and annotating the acute operating list for handover.

I've forgotten a pen, so I beg a spare one off Gaby. The hospital doesn't supply pens (even though they're essential for doing the job) and I've lost many of my own pens into general circulation. I have this theory that people in hospitals are either pen givers or pen receivers, and I am very much a giver.

The fishbowl starts to fill up with house officers and medical students. Our registrars arrive, drinking coffee. 'How are we looking?' they ask me, and I hand them a list. We're on two pages of patients, down from three the day before. Not bad.

Sam is rostered to a pre-admission clinic, so it's just me and Gaby today. Pre-admission clinic has to be my least favourite part of the surgical house officer job. In pre-admits, we see patients who are booked for elective surgery, who might have been on a waiting list for many months. Our job is to check that they are still fit to proceed for the surgery they've been waiting for, and to get any blood tests and investigations that are needed before the operation. Most clinics, I'll find someone whose surgery needs to be delayed. Sometimes we pick up a new heart murmur, or a new irregular heart rhythm. Often, we have a patient whose diabetes is so out of control that the risk of wound infections and poor healing would be unacceptably high. Once, I even diagnosed a broken rib in a patient who had fallen off his bike a week earlier and hadn't seen a doctor.

People waiting for orthopaedic surgery need it to help with severe pain, stiffness and loss of function. They are pretty gutted when I tell them they'll need to wait even longer until their new health problem has been addressed. Sam doesn't mind clinics and is good at them, so he picks up a few of mine, and I gratefully swap to look after things on the ward.

That day is the same as most of the others — not too busy, but not quiet. My team is a spinal team, with spinal injury patients who often stay in hospital for weeks or months and have frequent complications. One of them has pneumonia, and is getting better with antibiotics and chest physio. Gaby and I manage to get to the cafeteria before lunch is finished, and we exchange TV recommendations over our sushi. I've been rewatching *Critical*, a UK drama about a major trauma centre.

At 3 p.m. we run the list, figuring out what jobs are still left to do. A patient who has been very unwell with sepsis from multiple abscesses has a scan booked for 4 p.m., half an hour after our shift ends. I manage to convince Gaby to go home on time and let me stay and chase the scan, since she's just had a long day. It isn't always easy to convince Gaby to leave the hospital (although, in fairness, it isn't easy to convince me to leave either). We order blood tests for the next day. Gaby goes home, and I prepare a few discharge summaries while I wait for the CT result.

The CT report is uploaded at 5 p.m. It shows a new collection of pus that will probably need to be drained in the morning. I put in a theatre booking form, go through the surgical consent with the patient (who has had versions of this operation four or five times and no doubt has the spiel memorised), and I draw an arrow and my initials on his leg with surgical marker.

I get out of my scrubs, walk down the Rainbow Corridor, across the footbridge and into the parking building to my car. It's dark already, and cold. I start up the engine, turn on my audiobook and drive to the exit. I hold my parking card to the sensor. The display reminds me I don't have enough money on my card for the new weekly pass. Fuck. I push the button to call the parking office, but nobody answers. A car is approaching to join the queue behind me. I hastily reverse, and slip into a reserved park out of their way. I trudge back over the footbridge and across the road to the payment machine. I top up a few weeks' worth of my $12 weekly fee, and walk back to my car. Exit smoothly this time. The motorway is starting to clear, but the drive home still takes 45 minutes.

When I get home, I go straight into Charlie's study to say hello. She's working on an essay for her medical humanities course. I kiss her on the cheek, retrieve her empty mug from the desk, and head to the kitchen to put the kettle on. I make her an Earl Grey and set it down on the desk.

'Mm, thank you. Sorry, ten more minutes then I'll come out and start on dinner,' she says. I tell her not to be silly, that I can make it instead. It's not a particularly noble offer on my part; we've ordered My Food Bag this week, and the recipes are fast and easy. I potter in the kitchen, shaping little falafel balls and coating them in sesame seeds.

My mind wanders. I think about the elderly man in hospital with a broken hip, who is in pain and alone, with no next of kin. He told me today that he just wants to die. I don't know how you respond to something like that, so I didn't. I just squeezed his hand and sat with him in silence for a bit. Just before I left for the day I stopped by his room and he told me he remembered the name of his lawyer, who might be able to track down a nephew in Wellington. I'll try tomorrow.

Charlie comes out to the kitchen to help and I shoo her away. Dinner's almost ready. She turns on the news.

Over dinner, I ask her about her day. She begins the way she always does.

'So, I got up . . .'

Her classes have been online for most of the year, and her day is always the same. Boiled eggs for breakfast. A shower. A walk in the Domain and a takeaway coffee. Then ten or twelve hours at the little wooden desk in her study, fuelled by endless cups of Earl Grey. On a particularly exciting day, she might have spotted a new cat in the neighbourhood.

She asks about mine.

'It was good,' I say.

She rolls her eyes, like she does every day. 'Yes, but what happened?'

I grin apologetically. I'm terrible at recounting my day. At the end of my shift I can barely remember my name, let alone what I've done for the last ten hours.

'Well, I got up. I got my coffee and drove to work. Prepped the list. Did the ward round. Had a coffee. Did jobs. Oh, they've ordered butterfly needles for all the wards!'

Then I tell her I have a patient who has no family.

Vital Signs

'It's so sad. He's all alone. There isn't even anyone I can call to tell them he's in hospital.'

My eyes brim with tears, which eventually spill over.

'Oh, honey,' says Charlie, her voice gentle. She gives me her sympathetic smile and reaches out to touch my hand.

I try not to bring work home with me, but I don't usually succeed. I often think about my patients in my time off. Sometimes, if I'm really worried about a patient, I text the on-call doctor in the evening or over the weekend to ask how they're getting on. When they have left my care, or even when they have died, I find it hard to forget them.

After dinner, Charlie has more essay writing to do. She goes back to her study. I get into bed and watch *Brooklyn Nine-Nine*. It's the show I've seen ten times over and rewatch for comfort when I'm anxious or sad. Captain Holt's dog, Cheddar, has been kidnapped. Jake hatches a plan to pose as Holt's husband at the meet organised by the kidnapper. Next, Amy leads the precinct through a citywide blackout while in labour.

My best friend Wilbur texts me, asking if I want to get a coffee that weekend. Because of the pandemic he's home from Harvard and living in Auckland with his wife Prasanthi, but we've barely seen each other since I started on ortho. I'm working that weekend, so I suggest the following Sunday, which I have off. There's little use planning to catch up on a weekday evening: I never know what time I'll be done for the day, and even when I finish on time I'm not good company after work.

Charlie finishes up for the night at 9 p.m. By then, my eyes are heavy and my head is fuzzy. 'You okay if I watch something?' she asks, and I grunt my assent. She sits up in bed and watches an episode of some BBC miniseries. My early-morning starts have made me bad company, and I am usually half asleep by the time she has finished studying for the evening. I drift off to the sound of a suspect getting arrested by Nicola Walker, and sleep soundly until my alarm goes off again at 5.30 a.m.

CHAPTER 3:

The three Ps

YOU SPEND MOST of medical school learning about the human body, what can go wrong with it and how to treat it. You memorise the exact sequence of events that leads from HPV to cervical cancer. You can diagnose rheumatological conditions based on a single clue word in a question stem. By the end of six years, you think you're pretty clever. Then you start work, and quickly realise you know nothing at all about how to be an actual doctor.

I used to be an executive assistant at Parliament, which is a personal assistant to someone important enough that they give you better money and a fancier job title. I opened my boss's mail, answered his emails, organised his calendar and office budget, took minutes, planned events, did research and proofread documents. I bought his lunch while he was stuck in meetings, booked his hair appointments and picked up his dry-cleaning.

Most of my job as a house officer is just a better-paid, higher-stakes version of that. I print the patient list (basically the team's agenda for the day) and take the minutes on the ward rounds. My command of the photocopier is still my best asset, and my scary, professional phone voice still comes in handy when I need something urgently from hospital IT. I now order blood tests like I once ordered stationery, and arrange scans like I once made travel arrangements. Constituents concerned about 3G have been replaced with patients concerned about 5G, and emails have been replaced with discharge summaries. A good executive assistant knows everyone around Parliament, while a good house officer knows everyone in the hospital, and who to talk to so that things get done quickly.

The house officer is responsible for making sure that patient care runs smoothly, that investigations happen promptly, and that progress is documented. We need to know everything about our patients, starting with why they are in hospital and what needs to happen so they can be discharged. We need to know their medical history and living situation, how well they were managing at home before they were injured or became unwell, and how we think they'll manage now. We need to know what blood tests should be monitored to assess their progress, and what complications they are at risk of developing. We need to know who else is involved in their care, which might include family members, physiotherapists, occupational therapists, social workers, doctors from other services, or specialist nurses such as those working in diabetes or palliative care.

House officers should know what drains a patient has in their body and what is coming out of them, what other things we are monitoring (weight? food intake? fluid balance?) and how they are tracking. We know what antibiotics our patients are on and for how long, what their inflammatory markers are doing, and when they last spiked a fever. We should know if they have any electrolyte abnormalities, and should have done something to correct them long before the boss asks us. Every second person in hospital seems to have low potassium, and it feels like half the job is prescribing potassium replacement. We should know whether our patients are allowed to eat and drink and, if so, whether there are any restrictions (soft diet? clear fluids only? diabetic diet?).

We should know more than we probably ever wanted to about what patients' bowels are doing. When I was watching *Grey's Anatomy*, or when I was in my lab coat looking at pink and purple blotches through a microscope, or even when I was a student hunting the wards for willing prey so I could practise my consultation and physical examination skills, I don't think I realised just how much of my future day job would be spent thinking and talking about poo.

Some patients come to us with constipation, and some patients get constipation from us. Hospitals are not conducive to a good bowel habit. Strong pain relief, some anti-nausea medicine and even iron tablets can be wickedly constipating. One of the worst sins a house officer can commit is to chart opioid painkillers without also prescribing a laxative.

Patients in hospital are sick or injured, and not walking around much, which is one of the things that usually helps to keep us regular. They're also not eating their normal diet, and often they are sharing a toilet with three other people. It's a recipe for what we delicately call 'faecal loading'.

The nurses will ask every patient every day whether they've passed a bowel motion, and record it on a bowel chart. If there has been no luck, we step up the laxatives. We will try two or three different options orally, or 'from the top'. If it has been three days or more without a poo, we'll usually try 'from the bottom' and offer an enema.

If we often cause constipation in hospitals, the rest of the time we are causing diarrhoea. Sometimes we cause it with antibiotics, either the mildly annoying variety that stops when the course of antibiotics is finished, or severe and potentially life-threatening diarrhoea caused by infection with a bug called *Clostridium difficile (C. diff)*, which can overgrow when antibiotics kill off the normal good bacteria in the gut.

Liquid poo can even be a sign of severe constipation, called 'overflow diarrhoea'. This is when the hard lumps of solid poo are backed up inside, and the liquid poo behind them spills out, leaving the hard lumps behind.

Diarrhoea could be my fault, too, the result of overzealous prescribing of laxatives. Once constipation sets in, it can be hard to get things moving again without making things explosive. A favourite long-staying patient told me reproachfully on a ward round: 'Izzy, there is nothing less dignified than seeing your poo all over a nurse's uniform at three in the morning.'

The patients with diarrhoea get an isolation room and IV fluids. The patients with dark, tarry poo called 'melaena' (a sign of digested blood) get powerful antacids to protect the stomach, and a gastroscopy to look for the source of bleeding. Patients who aren't absorbing fats might have fatty poo called 'steatorrhoea' and need pancreatic enzyme replacement. Some patients come in with a change in their bowel habit or blood in their bowel motions. Those patients get a CT, and sometimes a colonoscopy, to look for inflammation or cancer.

On surgical wards, there is another reason to be obsessed with whether the patients have pooed. A fairly common complication of abdominal surgery is ileus, a condition where the bowel goes on strike, and the usual conveyor belt of poo pushed along by muscles in the bowel wall grinds to a halt. This leaves the gas, poo and digestive juices with nowhere to go, and they back up into the stomach, causing vomiting. The treatment for this is 'drip and suck': a plastic nasogastric tube down the nose and throat into the stomach. Nothing to eat or drink because it will just come up again, and IV fluids to keep on top of hydration and replace electrolytes. An ileus will get better with time, starting with a fart and followed by a poo. It is the reason we ask our postoperative surgical patients daily if they have farted yet, and celebrate when they have.

On television the first-year doctors are cutting surgical airways with a pocket knife, but in real hospitals we are booking a scan when the consultant tells us to. We all went into medicine to help people and to save lives, and of course we are still trying to do that, but most of the time, our contribution is paperwork, potassium and poo.

CHAPTER 9:

Responsibility

ALTHOUGH THE REAL medicine is mostly done by the grown-ups, being a junior doctor still comes with a lot of responsibility. The new responsibility can be terrifying. In your very last week as a medical student, when you are almost but not quite a doctor, you are not really trusted to do anything on your own. Discharge letters are checked and finalised by the house officer. The house officer countersigns anything you write in the patient notes. Your physical examination findings will be rechecked by a doctor. A few weeks later, after a brief holiday, you are a doctor.

When I first started, even the simplest task or the most minor decision took all of my concentration. I checked and double-checked every prescription. I ran even the smallest decisions past the registrar, afraid of inadvertently doing or saying the wrong thing. I would check our hospital handbook every time I needed to prescribe IV fluids. I would call another doctor for a second opinion on every ECG or chest X-ray. I would take a meticulous history from every patient I was called to see, even as the more mundane tasks piled up in my absence. The moderate confidence I had gained towards the end of medical school evaporated as my opinion and judgement suddenly had weight and consequence.

That terror made me safe, in a way. I checked and rechecked everything I did. It also made me painfully slow, which is its own kind of dangerous. Tasks sat on the Task Manager for hours while I was thoroughly investigating a headache for which I probably could have just prescribed some paracetamol.

I did make silly mistakes. Everyone does. So far I have been blessed that my mistakes have either been minor or have been caught early, and haven't had dire consequences. I have accidentally prescribed amoxicillin instead of amoxicillin and clavulanic acid, clicking the wrong thing in a drop-down menu while doing discharge papers in a hurry. I've prescribed an antibiotic without noticing that someone was allergic. I've also forgotten to sign prescriptions, and had to quickly scan and email a signed copy through to the pharmacy. The reason I haven't caused any harm, at least not that I know about, is because of colleagues who had my back: the community pharmacists who called me to double-check the medicine I wanted to prescribe; the other house officers who noticed that a discharge prescription looked odd; the nurse who called me to let me know about the patient's allergy.

Being a house officer also involves troubleshooting all manner of problems on the wards. Leaky IV line? Call the house officer. Difficult female urinary catheter that the nurses can't do? Call the house officer, who has done perhaps five female catheters in her life, but now needs to do this one. Drain needs removing? Call the house officer, who will look up how to do it on YouTube.

A medical degree gives you magic powers. For reasons that I will never understand, nurses are required to go on a special (and infrequently delivered) training course before they are allowed to do procedures like taking blood tests, inserting an IV line or a male catheter. These are tasks that could be taught to a layperson in an afternoon, certainly in less time than the three years of tertiary education completed by nurses before starting work. Many of these skills are actually taught in nursing school, and promptly lost when nurses start work and are not allowed to practise.

Doctors, on the other hand, learn these skills haphazardly in medical school and are expected to perform them competently on their first day on the job. For IV lines, our classmates were the victims of our earliest and most clumsy attempts. My friends and I would hide in the medical student room with a tourniquet, a sharps bin and a pile of cannulation equipment and insert and remove cannulae. Thankfully, we stopped short of inserting urinary catheters into one another. For that, we followed the 'see one, do one, teach one' approach.

After hours, when the bosses are at home and the registrars are seeing new patients in ED, it falls to the house officers to look after the patients on the wards. We answer calls from nurses who are concerned about patients, and need to be able to at least recognise if there is a serious problem, and call someone more senior in the (likely) event that we can't solve it on our own. I have lain awake after a long day into the wee hours of the morning many times, checking and rechecking in my head that I did everything right, that I had been a good, safe doctor during my shift. Did I read that ECG correctly? Did I rule out all the bad things that could have been wrong with that patient with chest pain? Did I remember to ask if the person with the headache had neck stiffness?

Some time during my final year as a medical student, I developed the habit of reading Health and Disability Commission (HDC) decisions. These decisions document the times when it has all gone wrong — when a health professional or the health system has failed to give someone the quality of care they should be able to expect, and they have come to harm.

In Aotearoa, blessed as we are in having ACC, lawsuits against doctors are rare, and we don't practise medicine in fear of being sued. However, we do have mechanisms including the HDC for investigating patient harm so that our system can learn from the cases, and if appropriate the people at fault can be referred for discipline by their professional body. The idea is to find out 'how could this have happened?' and to make sure it doesn't ever happen again.

There are an alarming number of ways in which you can harm a patient. You can forget to send a referral, or forget to follow it up, or not make it clear in the referral that the patient might have cancer and you really do need this CT urgently please, or not explain in the referral that someone is on blood thinners that they can't come off. You can prescribe the wrong medicine, or the wrong dose, or prescribe for the wrong patient. You can fail to recognise the signs of deterioration in a patient you are called to review, or fail to diagnose a problem correctly when a patient comes in to ED. You can kill someone by operating on them, or by not getting them to an operation fast enough. You can do all the right things for a patient, and then kill them by failing to hand over their care appropriately when your shift ends.

The system tries to mitigate this by having multiple layers of defence to stop us from killing patients. Prescriptions are reviewed by a clinical pharmacist, and blocked if they aren't appropriate or correct. Early warning scores calculated from vital signs help us to identify deteriorating patients, and empower nurses to ask the house officer to review, and to say 'They are scoring a six and need to be seen,' if they get any push-back. Electronic notifications tell us when there are new test results or scan results for our patients, and if there is something urgent then the lab or radiologist will usually notify the treating doctor by phone.

In healthcare we often refer to the 'Swiss cheese model' of protection, where there are multiple layers of defence against harm but each has some holes in it (like Swiss cheese). If the slices of cheese stack up in such a way that the holes are aligned, then harm occurs.

I dread creating a hole in a slice of cheese, being the busy junior doctor who failed to recognise the significance of a test result or who didn't order a test or scan that might have saved a patient. This is self-centred of me, but I do not know how I would survive knowing that I had caused a patient serious harm through my acts or omissions.

Fortunately, when you are a junior, the system protects you a little. Hospital policies prevent first-year doctors from deciding to designate a patient 'not for resuscitation', or altering a patient's early warning score so that an abnormal vital sign doesn't ring alarm bells.

House officers are taught to recognise when something is above our pay grade and to call a registrar for advice. Registrars run things past the consultants. By the time the buck stops with you, you have been training for over a decade. It is rare for the Health and Disability Commissioner to find against house officers because it is rare for us to have been the ultimate clinical decision-maker when a patient is deteriorating. When the Commissioner does find a house officer has failed, it is usually a failure to call for more senior help, or a failure of documentation.

In one recent decision at another hospital, the Commissioner made adverse comment against a house officer who had been told to monitor for deterioration in a woman with a massive pulmonary embolism, a blood clot in her lungs. The senior doctor in charge of her care had decided that at the time she was initially assessed, the risks of thrombolysis treatment outweighed the benefits. Thrombolysis is where a clot-busting drug is given that dissolves the clot but can cause internal bleeding. The senior doctor told the junior staff member that if the patient's systolic blood pressure was below 90 for fifteen minutes or longer, meaning that the clot was blocking the path of blood out of her heart so badly that she couldn't maintain effective blood flow to her organs, she would need thrombolysis.

A lot of other holes in the Swiss cheese lined up. She had low blood pressure, but an unidentified doctor in ED charted fluids to bring it up, presumably unaware of the reason it was low. Then the shift changed. The night house officer, responsible for every single medical patient in the hospital, was given a handover to keep an eye on her vital signs, and to call the registrar if they deteriorated. He was a second-year doctor, about as experienced as I am at the time of writing this. He checked her obs chart several times during the night, but didn't document that he had done so. A nurse contacted him with concerns that the patient was becoming more short of breath, and he reviewed her. The vital signs were stable, the blood pressure settled a little above 90. He discussed the patient with his registrar, whose opinion was that they should continue with the plan that had been made on arrival. The patient deteriorated further, and sadly did not survive.

The Commissioner was critical that the house officer had not documented his reviews, and had not called the consultant for advice. This case gave me a lot of pause, because truthfully I am not certain that I would have done things differently. I have certainly been guilty of forgetting to document that I have checked someone's vital signs, especially when they are stable or normal. Perhaps, if it was a quiet night and if we are being generous with me, I might have reviewed her in person and noticed the deterioration before it could be seen on the vital signs chart. But we do tend to trust our colleagues' judgement when their handover instructs us just to keep an eye on the chart, or to take action only if a vital sign deteriorates.

Would I have called a consultant in the middle of the night when the registrar was comfortable with the patient's progress and didn't want to change the plan? Probably not. That is above my pay grade, and I would definitely get told off for calling a boss at 3 a.m. Perhaps at my hospital, the involvement of the 'Patient at Risk' (PAR) team would have ensured that she received more senior attention earlier. Perhaps she would have been discussed at the 10 p.m. handover, and the admitting doctor would have told the night team he was quite worried about her, and that she would need to be seen in person. These are all good mitigations to have in place in a system vulnerable to human error.

Despite every mitigation, I am sure that I will one day be the doctor who makes the wrong call. In this job, your mistakes can matter. That is what keeps me awake at night. It is hard enough to bear witness to people's suffering, or to be the bearer of bad news. I don't know how I will handle it if I am the cause as well.

CHAPTER 10:

Breaking bad news

THE DAY BEFORE my last medical school exam, my dad called to give me the news that Granny Daisy had been in a car accident. She had fallen asleep at the wheel fifteen minutes from home, rolling her car down a bank beside a bridge, breaking both wrists, an ankle and the more trivial parts of the bones in her neck.

Dad is good in a crisis.

'She's going to be okay, but Granny has been in a car crash.'

I will always be grateful to Dad for the way he phrased that. I didn't have to wait a single second to know that she would be okay.

This wouldn't be a book about being a doctor if there wasn't a chapter about breaking bad news. There is something so profound and defining about being the person whose job it is to tell someone that they have cancer, or that a loved one has died, that I think it compels us to write about it.

In medical school communication skills class we are taught the 'right way' to go about it. Make time to sit down in a private room. Signal that you are planning to discuss something serious, and ask the patient if they would like their family to be present for the conversation. Even before that, signal what you are worried about.

'We are going to get an urgent CT scan. When we hear about your symptoms, especially for someone in their seventies, we are worried about cancer.'

Dr Chatterjee always introduced a possible worrying diagnosis with the same turn of phrase, one that I have borrowed many times since I started work: 'I'm not telling you this to scare you, but to be honest with you.'

Turn off your phone, or give it to a colleague. Bring a nurse, who will be left comforting the patient long after you have moved on to the next task.

Start by asking the patient what they understand about what is going on. This is useful information gathering, but is also a springboard into the hard part of the conversation. The part where you tell them the bad news, clearly and simply, without sugar coating.

'The CT showed that you have bowel cancer which has spread to your liver and lungs.'

That sentence might be the only one in the conversation they hear.

'When a cancer has spread like yours has, we cannot cure it, but some treatments may be able to slow it down. We would like you to see an oncologist about what treatments could give you some benefit, such as chemotherapy or radiation.'

Express regret that this is happening.

'I am so sorry to give you such bad news.'

Invite their questions.

'I know that was a lot of information. Do you have any questions right now?'

Sit with the silence for much longer than feels comfortable. If they have questions, do your best to answer them. If they don't, let them know that they will have more opportunities to ask questions. If they are crying, give them a tissue. Don't talk over them while they cry. Just wait.

As much as possible, avoid breaking bad news to patients when they are alone. If they are alone, ask if they would like you to help them tell their family.

Before you leave, make sure the patient knows the next step.

'The next step is to get a sample of the tumour in your bowel, by doing a colonoscopy. Having a sample helps us to make decisions about the best treatment options for you. That will happen later in the week, and we will tell you more about it tomorrow.'

We practise with actors, putting on our kindest faces and handing them tissues while they cry. We watch ourselves on video delivering bad news, and cringe at how awkwardly we try to offer comfort. Then, armed with all this new knowledge, we go out on clinical placements where we learn a hundred bad ways to break bad news.

In real life, patients learn of a new cancer diagnosis on the ward round while the patient in the next bed listens through the curtain. Patients are given bad news alone, and are then left alone. Patients wait for days to learn of their test results because it's a long weekend and the doctor on call doesn't want to tell them. Bad news is broken by rude doctors or busy doctors or doctors too junior to give useful answers to questions.

I will never forget, as a medical student, being sent to tell a patient that for another day running, the consultant wasn't in the hospital and so she wouldn't be told about her scan results. She asked me if I knew what the scan showed. I tried to think of how to answer without lying to her. 'I'm sorry, I really can't say.'

I knew the scan showed pancreatic cancer. She had come in sick and jaundiced and in terrible pain. She knew it wouldn't be good news. She knew it on the Friday when she had the scan, and on the Saturday, Sunday and Monday of the long weekend when she asked the on-call doctors for the results of the scan and was told to wait for her team to be back in the hospital. She knew it on the Tuesday morning when she'd been told to bring her family in for support, only to find out that the consultant was working at the private hospital and the registrar was busy in theatre, and finally, on the Wednesday afternoon as the registrar sat her down in the whānau room while I took notes, she knew for sure. She thanked him for letting her know.

On *House*, House describes his friend Wilson as someone people thank when he tells them they are dying. He means it as a signal of how nice Wilson is. Actually, in my experience a lot of patients thank their doctors for delivering bad news.

As a medical student, I found it hard to understand how the reality of communicating with patients could be so at odds with the methods we are taught. Had people only a few years further on in their careers really forgotten what they had been taught about doing this right? Worse still, had they forgotten their humanity?

As a still fairly fresh doctor, I now find it much easier to understand. At Middlemore Hospital you are hard pressed to find a private meeting room, with all available space filled up with as many patient beds as possible. Senior doctors busy in clinics and operating theatres have to delegate some difficult conversations to juniors. Jobs for the day fill up every bit of free space on the paper that holds my patient list, and my feet start to get a 'junior doctor itch' if I am in a patient's room talking to them for more than a few minutes. I catch myself feeling frustrated with someone who doesn't understand what I have already explained, rather than seeing it as an opportunity to help them to understand better. At 6.30 p.m. over dinner, a student nurse asks me what time my shift finishes, and I give her a tired smile and say '4 p.m.'

Sometimes I have to remind myself that a difficult conversation, the way I give upsetting news, is the most important thing I will do that day. Sometimes I have to remind myself to be a person.

I have broken really bad news by myself only a few times. I have called a family in the middle of the night to tell them they had better come in straight away. I have told women that they have miscarried, or that they have an ectopic pregnancy. Once, during lockdown, I had to tell a woman over the phone that her mum had died. It had been a difficult relationship, and they hadn't seen each other for many years, but she was still recorded as next of kin. What can you possibly say to offer a balm to the complicated feeling of losing an estranged parent? What can you say in the face of the grief at the relationship they had with them, and the better relationship they can now never have? I offered my condolences. She paused for a long time, then thanked me for letting her know.

In hospitals, you get a front-row seat to just how unfair life is, and your heart gets broken by it over and over again. You meet young people dying of cancer, old people dying before their kids can get home from overseas, and grumpy old bastards who smoke and drink, lie and cheat and still live to a hundred.

There is a superstition in medicine, at least half believed, that the worst things happen to the nicest people. As a medical student with time on my hands, I would spend ages talking to patients who were waiting for scans or to see the registrar in ED. I would build a good rapport, joking and bantering to make their stay in ED a little less miserable.

There is a moment, when you read the scan result of a

patient you've joked and bantered with, a patient you really like, only to see the worst news. Metastatic cancer. Probably only months. Your stomach falls through the floor. 'Damn,' says a nurse with more than a few grey hairs, looking over your shoulder. 'It's always the nice ones.'

You follow the registrar in to talk to them. They greet you with an enthusiastic smile, and you try to arrange your face into something kind and sympathetic, something a little more distant and removed than before. In that moment, you know that they are dying, and they have no idea. Perhaps they will be grateful that laughing with you distracted them from their fear and worry, at least for a little while. Perhaps you robbed them of an opportunity to prepare themselves, so that the news, when it came, was even more shocking. Perhaps it will all be such a blur to them that it wouldn't have mattered either way.

One of the first patients I admitted when I was a fourth-year medical student was a woman in her forties who hadn't opened her bowels in a week. She had a Kiwi accent broader than my Grump's, a daughter in her teens, and a mother who had died of bowel cancer. I liked her immediately, and stayed at ED until after hours to find out the result of her CT scan. It was bowel cancer, and it had spread to the liver.

When she got the news, she looked the registrar in the eye.

'Thank you for telling me. Could I please have a moment on my own?'

We left her to process it, all alone in a cubicle in the surgical assessment unit. I cried the whole walk home.

CHAPTER 11:

Ceilings of care

MODERN MEDICINE IS incredible. We can do supernatural things to keep a human body working when a part of it fails. When a young, fit and well person becomes very ill or injured, in a way that we think can eventually get better, we move heaven and earth to keep them alive.

If the blood pressure drops, we can give an infusion of a medication that artificially raises it. If the body stops moving air in and out of the lungs efficiently, we can put a tube down the throat into the airway and attach it to a ventilator. If the lungs temporarily stop working altogether, we can even oxygenate the blood outside the body. If the kidneys stop removing fluid and electrolytes from the body, we can attach a dialysis machine. If someone is unable to eat, we can put a tube into their stomach to feed them. If their intestines stop working and they can't digest food, we can give nutrition through an IV line.

We can support almost any failing organ in the body, at least for a little while. And because we can, the more difficult question becomes whether we should. A minority of the people who come to hospital are young, fit and well. For everyone else, we have to decide how much intervention is appropriate. We call this a 'ceiling of care'.

For people who aren't doctors and nurses, it can be hard to understand why there would ever be a limit to what you would do to save their loved one. Sometimes even when you are a doctor or a nurse it can be hard to understand why the ICU won't take the patient you have been working so hard to help. But over time, as you accumulate experience and watch a few people go through weeks or months of painful interventions and ultimately die anyway, it becomes easier to understand.

Patients who are so sick that they need their organ function replaced by machines suffer immensely. They suffer from their illness symptoms, which our treatments can alleviate, but can't take away completely, and they suffer from what we do to them. In the noisy ICU, a good night's sleep is nearly impossible, and the sleep deprivation will feel like torture. They have multiple tubes placed into their body. These hurt when they go in, and will restrict movement if they aren't already too weak to move.

If the tubes are in for long enough, there is a risk they will cause an infection, which means they'll need strong antibiotics. While bed-bound, their muscles will waste away from disuse. A previously fit, strong young man might become too weak for his legs to support his own weight. As these patients are unable to reposition themselves in bed unaided, nurses will have to do regular turns to prevent pressure sores, which might develop anyway. Being immobile in bed brings a high risk of developing blood clots, so we will give an anti-clotting medicine injected into the skin of the abdomen.

A young, previously healthy person going through a critical illness and needing ICU care suffers immensely, and still might not survive. Someone who started out elderly, frail and sick before the critical illness stands little chance of a good outcome if they deteriorate so badly that ICU would even be a question. All that ICU would add is suffering.

Doctors are taught four basic principles to analyse ethical dilemmas in healthcare. They are autonomy, beneficence, non-maleficence and justice.

Autonomy is the duty to respect the rights of patients to make informed decisions, and to decide what happens to their own body. This means that our patients get to decide that a stay in ICU or a big operation isn't what they want, even if we think it might be able to save them.

Beneficence is a doctor's duty to do good, and work towards getting the best possible outcome for our patients. This principle is easy for us: it is the one most of us had in mind when we started medical school. We wanted to serve others, to help people, to save lives.

Non-maleficence is the duty to avoid causing harm to patients. Don't operate on a patient if that operation will kill them. Don't bring a patient to the ICU if they stand no chance of survival, and if our treatments can only add to their suffering.

Doing good and doing no harm have been part of medical ethics for over 2000 years, and appear in the Hippocratic Oath. Autonomy is a newer principle, and it is sometimes the hardest one for doctors to swallow. It means that our patients might decide not to get the life-saving surgery or chemotherapy that we think is best for them. It means that our great ideas about how to prolong their life might not be what they want.

Justice refers to the fair and equitable allocation of limited health resources. This principle has always been in the background of decisions about treatment escalation, but it has been at the front of our minds during the pandemic, when doctors overseas have had two or more patients who urgently needed to be intubated and only one ventilator available, and had to decide which patient would definitely die, and which patient only might die.

There is no simple answer, and choosing the person in the best health to begin with, and who therefore might stand the best chance of survival, disadvantages people whose health has already suffered because of an unjust society.

Unless we screw up monumentally, nothing we do as doctors will make as big a difference to your health status as your education, ethnicity, and how much money you (and your parents) earn. We call these factors the social determinants of health. Access to clean water and a warm house that isn't overcrowded, a belly full of nutritious food so that you can learn at school, and the opportunity to focus on your education in your teens instead of working to support your family mean that you will, on average, have better health and a longer life than people without these things. If we choose to offer limited critical care resources to people who have better health, we are really offering resources to people who have had a more privileged life from the start.

When a new patient comes into the hospital, it is the job of the admitting doctor to start the process of thinking about the ceiling of care, and introducing this concept to the patient and their family.

The most basic form of life support is cardiopulmonary resuscitation (CPR). When a younger, healthy person's heart stops, there is a reasonable chance that the cause might be something we can fix, and that the heart might be able to get back to functioning well. When a frail, elderly person gets so ill that their heart stops, the chances of a good outcome are next to none. We can jump on the chest and give CPR, crushing until the ribs break. If we manage to get them back, the raw rib ends will grate together with every excruciating breath. Not being able to breathe deeply or cough will put them at a high risk of developing pneumonia. Their brain may have been without oxygen for long enough to suffer permanent damage. Their heart may have lost so much function that it fails, their body overloading with fluid that leaks into their lungs until they can no longer breathe.

Every hospital has some kind of resuscitation form that sits in a patient's notes to let staff know whether CPR is appropriate. At Middlemore this is a 'blue form'. If a person collapses without a blue form, the default for the nurses and house officers is to start CPR until a registrar can come to decide whether continuing CPR is appropriate. We want to avoid this uncertainty, so we try to make sure that every patient has a blue form.

Whether a patient receives resuscitation is not entirely up to the patient. Like other medical interventions, it is a patient's right to refuse resuscitation (in advance), but whether it should be offered is mostly up to the judgement of their doctors.

It's an awkward conversation to have. Many patients find the suggestion that their heart could stop a little confronting. A surprising number of elderly people and their families have never thought about it. Sometimes they feel blindsided by the question. Most people's experience of CPR is from television and movies, where people get a couple of shocks and make an immediate recovery without complications, so if CPR is not being offered, they struggle to understand why we don't want to save their loved one. 'We would like you to bring her back,' they often say.

Other people are more prepared for the possibility of their own death. 'If it's my time, you have to let me go,' one woman in her nineties told me, before getting better and going back to mow her own lawns at home.

Vital Signs

The other part of the blue form is whether someone is suitable for medical emergency calls, or so-called '777s', named after the hospital's emergency number. When a medical emergency call is made, usually because someone's vital signs are very abnormal, or because of a collapse or seizure, almost every nurse and house officer on the ward crowds to the patient's room. We are quickly joined by a medical registrar, ICU registrar and 'Patient at Risk' team of senior nurses specialising in resuscitation and the care of deteriorating patients. Often we will take blood tests, an ECG and a portable X-ray. We might put more IV lines in. We will measure the vital signs frequently, poke and prod and ask questions until we think we know what is going on.

This is a very good thing. It allows care to be provided rapidly for patients who need it, and gives the house officers and nurses some extra support when dealing with a clinical situation that concerns them. It is a good thing, but it is not the right thing for some patients. If a patient is dying, and the illness that they are dying from won't be reversed or changed by a 777 call, the disruption and discomfort of a 777 isn't a good option for them. In that situation, the goal of care shifts to comfort.

Of course, we don't always know. People we hoped might recover die in days. People to whom we gave comfort care and expected to die in days might recover and say hello to us in the supermarket months later. But for every patient who was given comfort care and lived, there are many more whose suffering could have been alleviated by reconsidering the goals of care, and who died.

There is a joke told to me by my friend Amber, an ICU nurse, which I have repeated to nurses at 2 a.m. on more than one occasion.

'Why do they nail coffins shut?'

'To keep out the doctors.'

We came into medicine to save lives. It isn't always easy to know when it is time to save someone's death. It isn't always easy to know when what you *can* do is different from what you *should* do.

Strictly speaking, ceilings of care and end-of-life matters are discussions that should be had with patients by registrars or consultants. Hospital policy protects house officers like me from having to initiate those conversations, but this policy isn't always reflected in reality. Sometimes the registrar is tied up at an offsite clinic or in the operating theatre, and the conversation can't wait. Sometimes patients and their families ask about it when nobody is around to defer to.

I've been called more than once after hours when a family member wants to restart active treatment on a patient receiving palliative care. There is no good way to have that conversation with a patient and family you don't know. If possible, it's a conversation that should be delayed until the patient's usual team is at the hospital. But on a Sunday morning, when the usual team won't be in for 24 hours and a patient's daughter is beside herself that we have stopped antibiotics and that every passing minute her mum's chance of survival is decreasing, there isn't much choice but to talk to her yourself. Anything else would be cruelty.

The most common reason for this situation is that a new member of the family has arrived, who wasn't present for the many conversations that happened leading up to withdrawal of treatment. Ideally, from the day the patient is first admitted, the admitting doctor has shared with the patient and their family that even with treatment, there is a chance they will not survive. Each day on the ward round, the team has told the family their impression of how their loved one is doing.

'Unfortunately, even with antibiotics, your mum isn't getting any better. Her breathing is becoming worse. We are worried that she might die from this illness.'

They will start to introduce the idea of shifting the goals of care.

'Your mum's IV line needed to be reinserted three times yesterday, which took many attempts. We are worried that treating her with IV antibiotics hasn't helped her get better, but is causing her suffering. How would you feel if we started focusing less on curing this illness, and more on making her as comfortable as possible?'

They will give the family time to think and talk about it, so that when the time comes to withdraw active treatment, it isn't a surprise.

'Your mum is getting more drowsy, and her breathing has been more difficult. I think that she is dying, and I want her to be as comfortable as possible. I think it's time to stop giving her IV fluids and antibiotics. We will give her strong pain relief, and medicines to prevent anxiety and agitation. How do you feel about that?'

The family members who have been involved in those conversations have had a little time to prepare themselves for what is to come. They have had the chance to ask questions. They have seen their loved one deteriorate day after day while still receiving active treatment, and they have heard the moans of pain from daily blood tests, tight blood-pressure cuffs, and pressure areas left on the face by high-flow oxygen masks.

When someone turns up who hasn't been having those conversations or seeing that suffering, it can be hard for them to understand why the doctors are doing this, and why their family members are letting it happen. Their loved one is dying, and they aren't even getting treatment! Their siblings or cousins are standing by and letting it happen! Not all families are close. Not all families trust one another to advocate well for a loved one. And sometimes it is just human nature to bargain in the face of impending loss.

In my mind, I am just a random house officer trying to get

Task Manager cleared before 10 p.m. handover. But to that family member, I am the doctor. I am the one gatekeeping the treatment that they feel sure will make their loved one better. So I talk to them.

I tell them I am so sorry this is happening to their mum. I ask them to explain to me what they understand about why she came to hospital, and what has happened while she has been here. Then I listen. They tell me she came in with a chest infection, and was getting antibiotics but now isn't getting any treatment. They tell me they've had no communication, and that the doctors have just decided to put their mum on the scrap heap. They tell me they waited hours until a doctor would even speak to them. If I can spare the time, I let them vent, try to let them have whatever catharsis they need.

Once they have finished, I tell them I am sorry, and I mean it. I tell them I know it must be incredibly stressful to have a loved one in hospital and not to know what is going on. Then I explain my understanding about what has happened. I try to summarise the days of ward-round conversations they missed out on.

'Your mum has been with us for just over a week. She came in with a severe pneumonia, and we started treating her straight away with strong antibiotics and IV fluids. We were very worried by how sick she was, and worried that even with treatment she would have a chance of dying from this illness. Over five days of receiving antibiotics through the drip, she kept getting sicker. Her breathing got worse and she started to get drowsy. She was showing us signs that we see in people when their bodies are starting to shut down. In talking with the rest of the family, we agreed that the most important thing for your mum now is to be comfortable. I am so sorry that you couldn't be here for those conversations. I wonder if, now that you are here, you have any questions about why this decision was reached, and what will happen next?'

Vital Signs

Most of the time, talking through the events of the admission is all it takes. It can be a great relief for people to know that we did everything we could, and that their loved one really was given the best chance of survival. Not all families are happy ones, and it must be awful worrying that your mum or dad's care suffered because a sibling you don't get along with was at the bedside instead of you. If, even after hearing about why the decision was made, someone is really adamant that they want to change the goals of care, I call the registrar. Those decisions and conversations are above my pay grade for now, and for that I am grateful.

CHAPTER 12:

Life

AS A JUNIOR doctor your life (or lack of a life) is dictated to you by the RMO unit (RMO stands for resident medical officer). The RMO unit manages the start paperwork, phones and tablets, rostering, sick calls and leave allocations of all the junior doctors in the hospital, as well as being a general first port of call for our gripes and questions.

A bad RMO unit makes life as a junior doctor impossible, or rather, they make it impossible to *have* a life as a junior doctor. Horror stories are whispered on the junior doctor networks of leave requests for doctors' own weddings, put in a year in advance, declined without recourse.

A friend of a friend reportedly overheard a staff member at an RMO unit training a new colleague, sharing the wisdom that 'you can't think of them as people'.

The staff in RMO units spend all day dealing with stressed, highly strung, type-A doctors, trying to convince us to work extra shifts to fill gaps in the roster. I am sure they are paid less than we are, and must roll their eyes a little when we try to negotiate a higher hourly rate for picking up a shift. I don't envy them the job.

A good RMO unit can make life easier for junior doctors. They arrange cover when we want to take leave so that our team isn't left in the lurch. They manage the resource of short-notice relievers who help out when a department is understaffed due to sick calls. They process our claims for additional pay when we pick up extra shifts, and our claims for public holiday pay and time in lieu.

The best ones even notice when someone is going to be the only house officer on a busy post-acute ward round, and recruit extra helpers from quieter parts of the service.

People generally suggest taking a week or two of annual leave every run to avoid fatigue. We are entitled to six weeks of annual leave a year, along with 30 days of sick leave. Like new parents with kids in daycare, new doctors get sick all the time. We are exposed to every lurgy circulating through the community. Even so, I have never met a doctor who came even close to using those 30 days of sick leave; before COVID, doctors generally worked through minor illnesses, and it is only the risk of transmitting COVID to patients that keeps us at home now. I think I have taken about five days off sick, almost all of them because I was waiting for PCR test results.

Between the long hours and the exhaustion, it's easy to become totally absorbed by medicine, especially when you are just starting out. Real life falls by the wayside. Exercise, hobbies and catching up with family and friends all give way to early ward rounds, late finishes, night shifts and double long-day weekends.

Like most new doctors, I find it hard to set a firm boundary around my personal life. I take on extra shifts when my department is desperate for cover. I worry about my patients when I'm at home, and sometimes if I'm really worried I log into my remote access to check on them. But the connections you keep to real life, and the non-doctor parts of you, are what keep you sane.

I'm ashamed to say that at times I take those things for granted. My family are mostly in Wellington or the South Island, and between travel restrictions and the demands of my roster I barely saw them at all during my first year. I managed to get some time off to go to Dunedin for my sister Georgie's law-school graduation, and to go home for Christmas. We fitted in family Zoom calls every month or so. My brother Harry was at Devonport completing his army training for some of my time in Auckland, and got to know Charlie over burgers and beers. My Aunty Alexis and Uncle Dave, and my cousins Josh and Aurelia, lived in Auckland with their big slobbering dog, Jess, and I visited them for dinner sometimes. I hadn't seen much of them when I lived in Dunedin, and in that time my cousins had turned from cute little rugrats to clever and insightful teenagers, who bantered gently with their parents and each other. I would sit on the couch with a herbal tea and smile as Aurelia teased her dad for taking too long in a shop, or Josh recounted a time when his mum had used her 'Karen powers' for good. Dave was a great gardener, and sent me home with a box of chilli plants for my flat garden.

The rest of my social life that year revolved around seeing colleagues at work, and my flatmates. In March, Paige joined us in La Roche. An accountant studying to be a psychotherapist, she is a little bit crazy in a lot of the same ways as Āria, Charlie and me, and we quickly became close friends.

We all made our way through *Legally Blonde*, *Practical Magic* and *Bend it Like Beckham* in our flat movie nights, and one weekend even convinced Paige to listen to our one-hour Taylor Swift Appreciation playlist, to get her to join us in liking Taylor's music. She maintained that it wasn't her cup of tea, but Ms Swift mysteriously made her way onto a few of Paige's

Spotify playlists. During lockdown, we bought a soccer ball so that we could kick it around in the Domain.

On weekends, Charlie and I would go to Daily Bread, where our favourite baristas Mitch and Jane knew Charlie by name, and quickly learned mine. Having a cafe where the baristas know your name is one of my most important measures of feeling at home in a new city. To our great excitement, one weekend when Charlie was away for the holidays and I was alone in Auckland, Jane told me that she and Mitch had started dating. I called Charlie the moment I got back to my car to tell her the news.

'Oh my god, two nicies together!' she said, and that became our nickname for the two of them.

In May, I turned 30. I decided to be brave and invite some people from work to my little birthday brunch at La Roche. Amber even came up from Dunedin. We made Bellinis with prosecco and blended-up canned peaches, and ate pastries from Daily Bread. Entirely characteristically, Gaby showed up, Brittany was on holiday that weekend, and Sam overslept.

In July, Wilbur and Prasanthi had a baby shower. We decorated onesies, competed in a quiz, and the stronger-stomached among us had a formula-drinking competition.

We spent most of the rest of the year in lockdown. In August the baby arrived, and I did a socially distanced placenta pick-up: for some reason it couldn't be stored at the hospital while Prasanthi recovered. Once the rules were relaxed to allow picnics, we went for walks with Gussie in the pram. Babies are not the biggest fans of masks, and he found my N95 a little alarming.

Sam came over for dinner one night and we had one of our signature rants about the state of the world, and some of the sad cases we had been part of at work. It was nice to be able to talk about work in an environment that was separate, and out of earshot of the people we were venting about.

I think doctors end up mostly being friends with doctors for good reason. The job can be incredibly isolating and lonely at times. We work unsociable hours and miss out on the important moments in our loved ones' lives because we can't get time off. We see a lot of really heavy things, things that are confidential and off limits when debriefing our days with our partners and friends. Our colleagues get it. They've cancelled their own plans at the last minute because of work plenty of times, and won't be offended if we have to do the same. They've been told off by the same bosses that we have, and can commiserate as we lick our wounds. We can talk shop to them without need for explanations.

But for the same reasons, it's important for us to keep in touch with our non-doctor friends. It's important to talk about something other than the hospital. That's a work in progress for me.

CHAPTER 13:

Diagnosis

WHEN I WAS in my teens, I called Healthline for some reason or other. I asked the nurse what she thought was wrong and she replied, 'Do you know what the two things are that nurses don't do?'

I didn't know.

'We don't diagnose, and we don't prescribe.'

That isn't true of all nurses these days — we have nurse practitioners and nurse prescribers who do diagnose and prescribe — but it does go some way to defining the role of the medical team.

We diagnose. We prescribe. We treat.

Diagnosis is the process of making sense of a patient's symptoms (what they tell you) and signs (what you see and examine), ordering test results and finally coming to a decision on the nature of the problem.

Every patient has pretty much one question: 'What's wrong with me, Doctor?'

Vital Signs

The two worst answers? Something. Or, nothing.

Nobody wants to have something seriously wrong with them. Obviously. They come to us worried because Dr Google thinks they have cancer, and they are hoping we will tell them they don't. What I think a lot of doctors find harder to understand is that it can feel just as much like bad news to be told there is nothing wrong when it *feels* like something is wrong.

When I was at university, I met Lucy. Lucy was an active, happy-go-lucky rugby player. Then one winter she slipped on ice on the way to uni, landing on her bum. After that, the pain started. Her legs started to give way. She had to walk with crutches, and could no longer play sport. She saw neurologists and orthopaedic surgeons, had X-rays and MRI scans, and finally, when every test came back normal, she was told that her problems were psychological. Overnight, she had become disabled, and the doctors could find no physical explanation.

Charlie has chronic back pain. There was no injury that she can recall, no single event that started it. She was a normal, healthy 22-year-old, and suddenly her back hurt. She tried stretches, strengthening exercises, yoga and pilates. She saw an orthopaedic surgeon, a musculoskeletal pain specialist, a chiropractor, an osteopath, a pain physiotherapist and a personal trainer. She has spent thousands of dollars trying to find out why her back is so sore, and trying to make it stop hurting. Her scans are normal, and don't explain the pain. Even if something was injured six years ago when the pain first started, that injury has long healed now, but the pain remains and her muscles have long since grown and wasted around the movement patterns she used to try to fix it. The pain makes it feel like something must be very wrong. It makes her wish she could put a knife or a hot poker in until she was pushing on the bit that hurt. Sometimes she touches the spot on my back that corresponds to her pain, perhaps trying to imagine what I must feel like with my pain-free spine.

Diagnosis

Just before I started medical school I sprained my ankle badly playing social netball. We were in the ladies' D grade, a team of Women's Refuge volunteers and assorted friends we had picked up during our two-year reign as the worst team in the league, our enthusiasm level high even if our skill level was low. That night we were winning for once. I was playing defence as always, and I collided with a shooter from the other team in the air, landing badly. The pain was so bad I couldn't walk on my foot at all. My teammates helped me hop off the court and down the stairs to my flatmate's car. I went to ED for an X-ray, but nothing was broken. I was sent home with crutches, paracetamol and an ACC brochure on self-care for my 'mild ankle sprain'.

I needed the crutches for six weeks. The first few weeks were the most painful, and between the sleep deprivation and the constant low-level ache I was exhausted and grumpy all the time. I saw a physiotherapist and did a million calf raises to strengthen the muscles that would protect me from further injury. I tried ice and heat, massage and compression. I went back to dance classes, doing what I could but avoiding any sudden changes of direction.

I moved to Dunedin and started university. I joined the gym and tried to get back into exercising, which had always been the best thing for managing my stress levels. I went to step classes, but each time my ankle was stiff and painful and I could barely walk on it for days afterwards. I went back to physio, but nothing seemed to help. I got referred to a specialist GP who could order an MRI. He asked me about my injury and examined my ankle. 'Ah yes,' he said, 'you have what I call a problem ankle.' I could have told you that, I thought to myself.

After the MRI, he said he wasn't surprised that it was sore. There was extensive scarring to my ligaments, but most importantly an area of the cartilage lining my joint had been sheared off by the impact, leaving the bone exposed. I remember feeling so relieved to hear this. Of course it was bad news that something was wrong with my ankle, but it was also validating. I was right: my pain was real.

I was referred to an orthopaedic surgeon, who offered me surgery that encourages a tough scar to form over the exposed bone. I jumped at the chance, and was on the operating table two days before my pre-med exams. I spent a long six weeks on crutches, and a longer six months avoiding high-impact activity like running and step class, but the operation was a success and my pain all but disappeared. I was fortunate to be in the minority of people with chronic pain whose pain could be surgically removed.

When she was in her forties, my mum became sick with a mystery illness. For most of my childhood she had been a supermum, making her six kids wholesome school lunches, running us between a billion extracurricular activities, keeping on top of the mountain of laundry, and having dinner ready on the kitchen table when we were all home each night. Suddenly she was so exhausted she could barely get out of bed. A former gym bunny, attempting to exercise made her sick for days, sometimes weeks. She felt a constant heaviness in her chest. Blood tests and an ECG were normal. She went to her GP many times over the course of a few months, but they could find nothing wrong.

After a year or so she got better, and for a few years she was well, back to being supermum. Then the sickness came back. This time she was diagnosed with myalgic encephalomyelitis/chronic fatigue syndrome (ME/CFS).

My mum's most extraordinary gift is that she is adaptable. I am sure she has grieved the changes in her life since she became sick, but as far as I can tell she doesn't dwell on that. She has goals in her career as a lawyer and local politician, and when she got sick, she found new ways to achieve her goals.

With a diagnosis came validation. A diagnosis meant community. It meant a reliable search term to type into PubMed on her endless search for new ideas to control her symptoms. She can often find a combination of supplements that helps for a little while, a few weeks or even months. Doctors are naturally sceptical of supplements, inclined to think they are sold for extortionate prices by people who make claims not backed by evidence. But can I honestly say that medicine has an alternative to offer that will work better than the supplements she has chosen to use?

When Mum was diagnosed, the medical profession's official answer to ME/CFS was something called graded exercise therapy (GET), which encourages sufferers to push themselves to do more exercise without regard for symptoms and adverse after-effects. This recommendation has now been officially withdrawn, partly in response to a campaign by members of the ME/CFS community, who say that the major study it was based on was flawed and did not consider the harm GET causes to sufferers of the disease.

There is often a tension between the medical profession and communities of chronically ill people, especially those with illnesses that are poorly understood by medical science, and especially illnesses suffered mostly by women. People want their doctors to be experts, I think, but they also want to be regarded as experts in their own bodies. With chronic illness, a lot of doctors let them down on both fronts. We lack expertise because something is rare or poorly understood, or simply because we have a bias against patients with so-called 'functional illnesses', where there is no identifiable cause or evidence on our tests and examinations. At the same time, we undermine the patient's expertise on their own body when we tell them that the tests are normal, that we cannot explain their symptoms or, worst of all, that nothing is wrong.

When I was at medical school I had lunch one day with a friend who was a medical sociologist. Conversation turned to chronic illness, as it often did: I have long been interested in the dynamic between doctors and the chronically ill.

'I just think,' I said over my roast-vege sandwich, 'that there is a violence in not being believed. I think that is why some sick people hate doctors.'

I was certain, in the way an eager young student often is, that I had discovered something profound. My friend smiled.

'Absolutely. There's actually a name for it — epistemic injustice.'

Of course someone cleverer than me had already thought of this, and had given it a name. Epistemic injustice. The idea that there can be an injustice in being treated as if you don't have knowledge that you actually do, and in having your experience dismissed.

A few years back on Twitter, a person with a genetic connective tissue disorder called Ehlers-Danlos Syndrome (EDS) started the viral hashtag #doctorsaredickheads. Thousands of people, mostly women, shared their experiences of being misdiagnosed, gaslit and dismissed when they took their chronic-illness symptoms to their doctor.

Medical school selects people who like to be good at things, and who like to be right. We were all the smartest kids in our respective classes. We want to do a good job for patients, but we also want to be thought clever by our colleagues.

Diagnosis is often hard. People come to us with a collection of symptoms and we try to make sense of them. We use diagnostic tests to discriminate between different problems with the same symptoms. We try to rule things in with tests that are only abnormal in certain conditions, and rule things out with tests that are rarely normal in certain conditions. The symptoms of chronic illness are often non-specific, overlapping with multiple other physical and mental health concerns.

Our training teaches us to prioritise the objective, what we can measure and observe, over the subjective, what the patient feels. The objective sometimes disproves what the patient tells us. They felt like they had a fever, but had a normal temperature and normal blood tests when we saw them. They felt like they had blurred vision, but on examination could see normally. They told us they had ten out of ten on the pain scale, but were observed using a cellphone. (That a person truly in pain doesn't use their phone, or indeed do anything other than lie with their eyes shut looking sore for the benefit of doctors, is one of my very least favourite ideas in medicine.)

There is a whole group of ailments that we group together and collectively call 'medically unexplained symptoms' or 'functional symptoms'. Problems with the body's function, when we can find nothing wrong with its structures. Subjective symptoms in absence of objective proof. Chronic pain that doesn't represent any ongoing injury. Seizure-like episodes that are not caused by epilepsy. The inability to speak or walk when nothing is structurally wrong. Psychosomatic symptoms or conversion disorder, where stress or distress is converted to physical symptoms. The sufferers of this type of ailment are disproportionately women, and young women especially.

Diagnosis can be a double-edged sword. A label can validate a patient's symptoms, help them to understand what is happening in their body, and make them feel less alone. Having a name for what is wrong can mean freedom from searching for answers that might never come. It can also mark a patient as someone not to be trusted, someone whose pain is less likely to have a worthy explanation, someone who is probably making this up. It must be horrible to be told that your suffering is in your head. People with psychosomatic or functional symptoms are not faking their symptoms, and their pain and distress is real, but it's hard to differentiate being told that your mind is causing your symptoms from being told that you are faking it.

Doctors can find this distinction hard too, I think, and these diagnoses tend to carry a degree of stigma in the medical community. I think on some level a lot of doctors believe that if the patient says they have symptoms but our tests say there is nothing wrong, it must be the patient who is wrong. Sufferers are sometimes labelled 'heartsink patients', to whom we have little to offer, and their (often multiple) diagnoses are recited with the implication that whatever new complaint we are seeing them for must be in their heads as well.

I am counting myself in this. I would love to think that I am or will be a doctor who always takes people's symptoms seriously, who doesn't let my bias impact the care I give my patients, and who believes people's accounts of what is happening to their own body. I would love to think I am one of the good ones. But I trained within the same system as everybody else, and grew up in the same society. I have the same tendency to dismiss and disprove.

I think every doctor believes themself to be one of the good ones, and in doing so we give ourselves a free pass. As long as we are one of the good ones, we don't have to think too hard about which patients we take the most seriously, which patients we roll our eyes at, and where that distinction might come from. As long as we are one of the good ones, we get to leave our biases unexamined.

CHAPTER 143

The empathy exams

THE DAY I moved from Wellington to Dunedin to start medical school, Wilbur gave me a printout of an essay by Leslie Jamison from her book *The Empathy Exams*. It is a story of her time as a medical actor for medical student exams, marking students against a checklist for their wooden displays of empathy. 'That must be really hard,' they would all say, as her character shared the loss of her brother, and the seizures that had started afterwards. It is also a story of her abortion and her heart surgery, and an exploration of empathy, which she describes as 'perched precariously between gift and invasion'.

When I began medical school, I was delighted to find that the exams described in the essay really happened. We call them 'OSCEs' (pronounced 'oskies'), which stands for Observed,

Vital Signs

Structured Clinical Examinations. In this type of examination, students either take a history from or perform a physical examination on an actor, while being observed by between one and three senior doctors.

In the earlier years of med school, we do this once a year, with a whole year of 'clinical skills' tutorials leading up to a 30-minute exam. My tutor is Linda, a senior ICU nurse with a few decades of experience who is as proud as a doting parent when we do well.

We learn the Calgary-Cambridge model of history-taking, where we open the session by finding out what problems the patient has been hoping to discuss with the doctor, and what they would like to talk about first. Linda tells us she once asked a patient, 'So, what's brought you in here today?' and got the answer, 'I walked.'

We learn to gather information on symptoms. For pain, we learn the SOCRATES framework, asking about the site, onset, character, whether the pain radiates, associated symptoms, time duration, exacerbating and relieving factors, and severity out of ten. We start to learn the clusters of symptoms that point to a particular diagnosis. At the start of medical school, our job isn't to know what is wrong, but it helps to know what symptoms to ask about.

On exam day we stand outside a tutorial room, reading a brief scenario as the timer counts down.

> *You are a medical student attached to a General Practice. Ms Anita George, a 37-year-old practising lawyer, has made an appointment with her GP spurred on by a comment from a work colleague suggesting she might have a drinking problem. Your task is to begin to explore the nature and extent of Ms George's alcohol use and build rapport with her. You have seven minutes to complete the station. After six minutes*

*there will be a one-minute warning. You should
conclude the interview in the final minute.*

The timer goes. We knock, and enter our rooms.

Anita George is a successful lawyer who owns her own
practice. Her work can be stressful, and she uses alcohol to
cope. She is elegant and well dressed (the actors are under
strict instructions not to look shabby), enjoys tap-dancing and
old movies, and her drink of choice is Central Otago pinot noir,
which she orders online. She drinks two bottles of wine every
night, and feels sick if she takes a night off. Both her parents
were alcoholics, and died when she was in her twenties. She
has no siblings. She is single, has no children, and no flatmates.
She is all alone.

The actor playing Anita has been instructed to give very
limited information unless the student shows an effort to build
rapport, and makes an attempt to understand her situation
non-judgementally. Out of twenty possible marks, twelve are
for communication skills: opening the consultation, rapport-
building, asking questions effectively, exploring Anita's
perspective on her drinking, and making the actor feel listened
to and understood.

The rest are for garnering specific pieces of information about
her drinking. How much, and how often? Does she ever have
days without alcohol? Over time, has she needed more alcohol
to achieve the same effect? Has alcohol caused problems at
work, or in her relationships? Does she ever take risks while
drinking that she wouldn't take sober: driving drunk, risky sex?
Does she black out? Is she depressed? Does she suffer from
anxiety? Is she using other drugs besides alcohol?

The same pool of actors is used for training scenarios and
exams for the five years of medical school. The woman who
wanted to hide her chlamydia from her husband now has a
busted knee from playing rugby. The teenager whose mum

was worried because he stayed up playing video games and could never get up in time for school is now 25 and has blood in his stool. The older man who probably had bowel cancer now probably has lung cancer.

We run scenarios dealing with angry, frustrated patients, patients whose appointment started 45 minutes late and who don't think they should have to take time off work to see a GP every six months to get the same inhaler they've used for five years. We practise breaking the news to a woman that her husband has died unexpectedly of a surgical complication. We speak with a patient so depressed she can barely speak. The actor slows her speech and movements down, in the way they are slowed when someone has severe depression, and we feel the energy drain from our bodies as we speak to her. We talk to a young woman who has impulsively taken an overdose after a fight with her boyfriend.

We get used to being recorded on video showing empathy for all this false pain, or false representations of pain that has been real for someone, sometime. We watch back and dissect our body language and the words we used. Did I leave enough silence? Did I reach out to touch their arm sympathetically? Did my expressions of empathy sound natural, or rehearsed and wooden? Did my naturally expressive face and clear, earnest voice come across as condescending?

The idea of all this practice is that by the time we are doctors, we will have some skill in the art of medicine, as well as the science. It will mean we can bear witness to the hardest moments of other people's lives, and respond the way a good doctor would.

The Empathy Exams was the start of my obsession with medical creative writing. I have gravitated ever since towards reading and writing essays about being a doctor or being a patient. Another favourite is 'Medicine's uncanny valley: the problem of standardising empathy' by Caleb Gardner, an essay published in *The Lancet*. Caleb was a medical student when his father died of heart failure, and the essay explores how it felt to be on the receiving end of insincere, scripted empathy from one of his father's doctors.

I started working as a doctor at age 29, six years older than my youngest colleagues, but still feeling far too young and too awkward to do this job. My life has not been completely sheltered, but it has still been one of relative privilege.

I am still learning the right things to say on days when there is nothing 'right' to say. I am still learning to hold space for people on their worst days, when they have received the worst news, and even when they are their worst selves. Sometimes all I can give is my silent company. Sometimes all I can give is time to themselves. Sometimes my empathy slips out unfiltered. 'I'm so sorry, it's really shit.'

I don't understand how most of my patients feel, at least not yet. In time, I am sure that I will. Being well and able-bodied is temporary for all of us, and we will all have an experience on the other side of the line between doctors and patients.

One normal day in med school, my friend Julia and I were sitting in the lounge with her flatmates watching *MasterChef*. We were snacking on a cheese platter, sipping pinot gris and swooning over Melissa Leong's earrings.

Julia's phone rang and she left the room to take the call. That wasn't unusual: her parents called her most days. We continued watching Melissa as she tasted contestants' dishes, never once ruining her lipstick or splashing sauce on her dress.

Julia returned and sat back down. Melissa gushed her heart-felt praise for a contestant's dish that spoke to their heritage, and we all swooned. The show finished and we chatted for a while longer, lingering over the last few sips of wine and cutting ever smaller slices from the remaining wedge of cheese.

Then, in the comfortable silence that followed, Julia spoke.

'So, about the phone call I got before,' she said, not looking at anyone. 'My grandad's had a stroke.' Her voice was even and factual, the way it always is when she talks about upsetting news.

Julia's grandfather, Jack, is in his eighties, and over her time at medical school his health has declined in the way that so often happens with people in their eighties: they slow down gradually and insidiously, able to manage a little less every day, until one day you are helping them to the car and it strikes you that they are old. Except that now it had declined suddenly, and all at once.

He had been at home by himself, as he often was during the day. His wife, Barbara, a few years younger than him and in better health, enjoys going out to play bridge, so things had been set up at home to allow Jack to manage independently during the day. He had a freezer full of ready meals to put in the microwave, or ingredients for simple meals like bacon and eggs that he could make for himself. He had only recently stopped driving, and when he could drive he had spent his days at his favourite neighbourhood cafe eating club sandwiches and catching up with friends.

When Barbara arrived home he was sitting on the couch, as he often did. She greeted him and set about cooking dinner. When it was done, she called out to him that dinner was ready. He didn't move.

'Are you coming to the table?' she asked.

'I can't,' he said in his lilting Irish accent. 'I've had a stroke.'

Several hours earlier he had suddenly developed a splitting headache and lost the use of his right side. He hadn't pushed his St John Medical Alarm to call an ambulance. Julia suspects he felt that calling an ambulance would make it real. She thinks he wanted his life to stay the same for just a little while longer.

For some strokes, a few hours can make the difference between treatment and no treatment. The doctors said that wasn't the case for Jack. He wasn't a good candidate for clot-busting treatment, and he wouldn't have been offered it.

It was scary and strange being on the other side of healthcare, even indirectly. When you have a loved one in a hospital in another city, it's nearly impossible to find out what's actually going on. It's hard to get the doctors on the phone and, unless the person in hospital (or their support person) is medical, they don't always come away from the morning ward rounds having absorbed and understood everything that was said.

Having been on both sides, I understand why updates aren't given to families every single day. A lot of the time, from a medical point of view there is no real update. The plan is the same as before, and there is no particularly important progress to report. The ward-round note reads:

> *Imp: stable*
> *Plan: cont*

But being on the other side feels absolutely horrible. You have no idea what's going on, and you don't really have anyone to ask. Julia's mum has a busy job and couldn't always be at the hospital, and Julia herself is the only medical person in her family, so she went home so she could spend all day at Jack's bedside.

She crammed for her next exam in the two days spent sitting at his bedside, and still got an A.

While Jack was still in the acute stroke unit, the nurses accidentally dropped him onto his paralysed arm. They obviously didn't think much of it, and it wasn't reported. The next day, when Julia went to see him, he kept complaining of pain in his wrist, and he told her that the nurses had dropped him. She was worried, and since there wasn't a doctor available she examined the wrist herself. When she did, she became more convinced that there might be a problem. She asked the nurse to call for the house officer, and asked if he thought her grandad might need an X-ray. The scan showed that he had broken a bone in his wrist and would need to spend the crucial first few weeks of his stroke rehab in a cast.

Julia is a gracious soul and she isn't angry that the nurses dropped him. Lifting people is hard, and accidents happen. But I can't help wondering whether anyone would have noticed Jack's broken wrist if his granddaughter hadn't been a medical student.

Before too long, Jack transferred to a rehab ward to start the long process of recovery. His wasn't the worst stroke, as strokes go, and his rehab went fairly well. His right arm doesn't do much these days, but his legs can do a little more. He can walk a short distance with his walking frame and a little help. He can understand what people are saying to him, and he can speak and make himself understood. But every small thing is a huge effort now, and it wasn't before.

After months of rehab he was ready to be discharged from hospital. The geriatrician told Julia and her mum that Jack was probably in need of hospital-level care, which would be difficult for Barbara to provide at home. Barbara was pretty well for her age, but still in her late seventies, and lifting Jack would be hard work. But she wanted to try, and the hospital supported them in that. Arrangements were made for them to have care workers in twice a day to help with tasks that were too heavy for Barbara to do alone: getting him up, showering and toileting.

Caring for another human full time is hard enough (or so I'm told) when it's a 15 kg child. It's harder still when it's a 60 kg man who sometimes gets confused, and needs to take medication several times a day.

The carers were nice, but unreliable. This wasn't the fault of the individual carers, but of the agency that allocated their tasks for the day. At the best of times, you never really know what time carers are going to show up, and can't easily plan to do anything outside the house in case they arrive while you aren't home. But more often than not, short staffing meant that no one came at least one of the two times they were due each day. They never called to tell Barbara this: she would simply wait, having delayed any plans to go out so that she would be home when they arrived, but they never came.

The rest of the year was hard for Julia. She didn't want to withdraw and have to redo the whole year, so she came back to uni to continue studying, but she was worried sick about her grandparents. She planned to drive the few hours home as often as she could in between compulsory classes and exams, every weekend if she could manage it. Then, a week after Jack was discharged, COVID reached New Zealand, and travelling was no longer an option.

Julia's whole family are incredibly proud of her achievements, and are so excited for her to become a doctor. They shielded her as best they could from the realities of how hard it was managing her grandad's new disability at home, and it wasn't really until she went home for the mid-semester break that she saw how difficult life had become. Barbara had made it to bridge only a few times in months. She was exhausted, and had badly injured her back lifting Jack when the carers hadn't shown up. Julia's mum and brother went around to help out as much as they could, but they had jobs of their own.

Julia's plans for an overseas elective were foiled by COVID and she chose a research project she could complete remotely. She went to stay with her grandparents to give Barbara a little respite. She could go to bridge or get a coffee or a glass of wine with her friends without feeling guilty, and without needing to find an adult 'babysitter'. On days when the caregivers came, she didn't need to help with lifting at all. On days when they didn't, she found her back was so sore that she couldn't really help anyway.

Caregiving can be lonely work. There can be a lot of love in gently and carefully looking after a loved one's basic needs, but it can also be isolating. Julia could go out to see her friends sometimes, but she had to plan carefully so that her grandad would be looked after. Even when she did go out, she felt a little separate from her friends, who had never been carers.

By the end of Julia's elective it was becoming clear that Barbara looking after Jack at home wasn't going to be sustainable long term. Short staffing at the carer agency was at crisis point, and there were more days without any carers than days with them. Seven months after his stroke, and four months after he had been discharged home, they came to terms with the need for Jack to go into care.

If you, like me, have been blessed by not yet being required to put a loved one in care, you might think that with the decision made, things would become simpler. But it took weeks and weeks to find a home that had space, and once he had moved in, the visiting hours and COVID restrictions made it hard to call on him often, and his declining mobility made it hard to take him on outings.

Watching what Julia and her family went through in the months following Jack's stroke made me wonder about all the elderly people I had seen being discharged home with 'increased supports'. I wondered if their carers were showing up. I wondered if the equipment they were promised ever arrived. I felt naive for never considering this before, and for assuming that because those things were supposed to happen, they actually would. I wondered what happened to the people who had nobody to look after them, and who couldn't get out of bed without the help of their carers. Did they just stay in bed if no one showed? Did they have no choice but to soil themselves, and wait for it to be cleaned up the next day?

Because of Jack and Barbara, I will always take a few extra minutes to find out how my older patients are really managing. I don't just assume anymore that the system will catch them.

CHAPTER 15:

Medicine

IN JULY, AFTER a long three months of looking after broken bones and spinal injuries, I moved on to my rotation in general medicine. Gen Med is where patients go when they have some of the most common reasons for hospital admission — including pneumonia, heart failure and chronic obstructive pulmonary disease (COPD) exacerbation — or when they don't yet have a diagnosis.

Gen Med was my only first-year run without another house officer on the same team. I was on the same ward as Brittany and another colleague from ortho, so at least I would have someone to get coffee with.

We were on Ward 17, miles away from the rest of the medical and surgical wards, in the same building as the maternity wards. It was a small and poky ward with very few private rooms, the most irritating call-bell sound I've ever heard, and a tiny office where too many staff shared not enough chairs and computers. There were only two saving graces. The first was a huge lolly jar refilled weekly by one of the medical consultants. The other was the excellent nurses.

Perhaps because the ward was so challenging and so far away from everywhere else, they had cultivated a staff of very switched-on and dedicated nurses, and had trained them well. They knew all the patients on the ward at any given time, even the ones they were not personally caring for. They were particularly skilled in palliative care, and would help me when I felt out of my depth caring for people in the last days of life. Several of them were trained to do bloods and put in IV lines, which avoided delays when the after-hours phlebotomists and on-call house officers didn't want to walk all the way to the ward.

Middlemore Hospital's medical teams are named for native trees. I worked on the Kauri team, while Brittany was the house officer for Tītoki. Every morning at 8 a.m. the huge department would gather in a big meeting room to make sure all the new patients were assigned to a team, and to even up the workload for the day.

The registrars and house officers whose teams were post-acute would have arrived early to look up the patients on the list, checking for readmissions best looked after by their original team, and for people who might be better cared for under one of the medical specialties. We also had to check that all the new patients on our list were crossed off a giant reconciliation list at the front of the room, which listed every medical patient admitted in the last 24 hours, to make sure nobody was missed.

Handover started with a report on any patients who became sick or died overnight, which I mentally nicknamed 'the sick and the dead'. The night team would then mention by name and diagnosis every patient who had been admitted overnight. Teams would ask specialty registrars if they were willing to see patients, and hand back to their original team any patients readmitted less than two weeks after being discharged. New patients who had popped up on the list of a team that hadn't been on call would be reassigned to a post-acute team.

A couple of times a week, the handover meeting would finish with a brief teaching session by one of the consultants. One of them, Dr Shaba, had an acronym for virtually every topic in medicine, and could whizz through one on the whiteboard in ten minutes.

Side effects of clozapine (a medication used in treating schizophrenia):

CLOZAPINE

C	Carditis, constipation
L	Leukopenia
O	Obesity
Z	Zzzzzzz . . . sedation
A	Agranulocytosis
P	Postural drop of blood pressure
I	Increased heart rate
N	Neuroleptic malignant syndrome
E	Embolism (pulmonary)

Medications that cause low sodium (hyponatraemia):

LO SALT3

LO	Losec (omeprazole, and other proton pump inhibitors)
S	SSRI antidepressants
A	Antipsychotics
L	Lamotrigine
T3	Tricyclic antidepressants, tramadol, Tegretol (carbamazepine)

Vital Signs

These mini teaching sessions were the best part of the day. They reminded me of being in medical school on Dr Chatterjee's Gen Med team, where I learned more than in any other rotation. Dr Chatterjee has won several teaching awards, and would give impromptu tutorials to the whole team on quiet afternoons. I finished my degree with a very rosy view of Gen Med, and thought for a while that it might be what I wanted to do forever. Of my four first-year runs, it was the one I was the most excited for. That excitement quickly dissipated.

Gen Med at Middlemore is a notoriously brutal rotation. The patient numbers are high, and the patients are often very sick and very complex, with a large number of what we call 'comorbidities' — chronic health conditions that coexist. Some weeks there are three post-acute days, and new patients are admitted long before old patients can get better and get discharged. We send patients home without discharge papers while we're on the ward round so that a bed isn't blocked by someone who doesn't need it, then have to stay at work late to catch up on all that paperwork.

My team seemed to get a lot of patients with social complexity and barriers to discharge, either through luck of the draw or because historically our 'home ward' had specialised in looking after these patients. This meant that a lot of patients on our list would be with us for weeks at a time, acquiring further complications from being in hospital while we tried to figure out how they could be safely discharged.

Being a medical house officer was a huge adjustment. After three months in orthopaedics I had felt like a good house officer. The pattern of how orthopaedic problems are managed and how patients usually recover became familiar enough that I could predict what investigations and management the seniors would order. I got used to managing the same few after-hours ward calls again and again. The nurses learned to trust me, and even like me. I had become fairly confident in keeping track of my patients' bloods and vital signs, and managing the non-bone-related aspects of patient care, such as electrolyte abnormalities, urinary tract infections, deteriorations in kidney function and chest infections. I called for advice if I needed it, but could also solve simple problems myself by using my knowledge and research skills or following hospital protocols. By the end of the rotation I (sometimes) felt like a doctor.

In Gen Med, almost all the decisions are made by a registrar or above. Medical registrars spend more time on the wards with their house officers than surgical registrars do. They do still have other responsibilities, going to clinics and admitting new patients in ED, but at least a couple of days a week they are around the wards helping with ward jobs. This is a very good thing because there are a lot of ward jobs, and a lot of sick patients, but it does mean that during normal business hours house officers are mostly secretaries, and are not really expected to do very much on our own. Even the laxatives were often a registrar decision.

Medicine was a weird and lonely rotation for me. A couple of weeks in, my usual reg, whom I really liked, was redeployed to the COVID ward, and one of my two bosses had to switch to doing non-face-to-face work because of COVID. I had many different relievers for the rest of the run, some for a few days at a time, some for up to two weeks. They were all great doctors, and all very nice to me, but they didn't know me and so understandably didn't trust me to do anything. Our patients on Gen Med were also very sick. A long stayer I liked a lot died suddenly one weekend when I was on call, which hit me hard.

Through the ups and downs of psychiatry and the early morning starts of orthopaedics, I had always basically liked being a doctor. During Gen Med, I was bored and miserable. I found it nearly impossible to drag myself out of bed for work.

I looked forward to night shifts because they meant I wouldn't have to do a ward round or stay late doing paperwork. On night shifts, when things weren't too busy, I would sit and chat with the nurses on Ward 17. They always had the best gossip, and knew all the dramas going on in the hospital. Through them, I would hear which doctors and nurses had started dating, which consultants had been in trouble with the head of department, and which ones had been deemed so mean that they were banned from having students.

When things were busy on nights I diagnosed myocardial infarctions and pneumonia, treated fluid overload with diuretics and dehydration with fluids. Unlike during the daytime, on nights I got to be a doctor, and I did learn a lot. Gen Med made me a better doctor. It just made me really, really miserable too.

CHAPTER 16:

A mind stretched

EARLY ON DURING Gen Med, my consultant bought me a coffee and mentioned that she'd noticed I looked stressed out and unhappy on ward rounds. I apologised, and explained that I had become used to the short ward rounds of surgical teams, which leave most of the hours of the working day free to do 'jobs' — ordering scans, chasing results and speaking to other services for advice. I was worried about getting everything done.

What she told me then has replayed in my mind many times since.

'My ward rounds are long,' she told me, 'and I know that can make your day busy. But it would be unacceptable to me if a patient came through this hospital under my name and never understood what we thought was wrong, and how we treated it.'

This happens all the time in hospitals. It happens even when we think we've explained things fairly well, maybe even think we've put extra time into sitting and talking with the person to make sure they understand.

The Middlemore learning centre, Ko Awatea, is three quarters of the way along the Rainbow Corridor. Like many adult learning environments, its walls are adorned with quotations about learning. One quote, attributed to Oliver Wendell Holmes, has always jumped out at me: 'The mind, once stretched by a new idea, never returns to its original dimensions.'

I think of that not so much as an aspiration but as a caution. I have now studied one year of basic sciences, two years of pre-clinical medical theory, three years of clinical medical school, and one year as a doctor. I didn't do biology in high school, and in my first few months of pre-med I learned what a cell was, found out that kidneys make urine, and learned that nerve impulses are a form of electricity. But more than just knowledge (which is easily forgotten), my training has instilled an intuition for how bodies work, and an ability to recognise patterns in the ways that their function can fail. My mind has been stretched a long way in one direction, wrapped around organ systems and homeostatic mechanisms until thinking of them isn't a stretch, but a resting position.

One of the most common reasons people come into hospital under Gen Med is for what we call 'decompensated heart failure' — when the heart is not pumping as well as it should. It is the job of the heart to pump blood to the lungs to pick up oxygen, and to the rest of the body to deliver the oxygen where it is needed. When the pump is not working very well, blood backs up, and the extra pressure causes fluid to leak into the lungs and the legs. Fluid in the lungs makes people breathless, especially while lying flat (when gravity lets the fluid accumulate). Treating this involves giving diuretics so that the extra fluid comes out as urine. We also restrict water intake to prevent more fluid from building up, and weigh the patient daily to track progress.

'Your weight has gone up 8 kg since last month, so we are going to need to give you some powerful diuretics through a drip,' we tell them on ward rounds. Over and over again, I listen to patients apologise ruefully that they have gained weight. 'I didn't get out for enough walks over lockdown. I've been eating too many takeaways.'

Later, when I have a bit of time, I come back to explain.

'Weighing you isn't about finding out if you're fat or skinny. The reason we do it is because at the moment you have too much fluid in the body. A litre of water weighs one kilogram, so the most accurate way we can tell how much extra fluid we need to get rid of is by weighing you.'

For many patients I am not the first doctor who has tried to explain their condition, and I am sure I won't be the last. There are days when I have spent what feels like a long time painstakingly explaining something, printing out patient information leaflets with diagrams and answering any questions. Then when my reg or consultant talks to the same patient on the morning ward round the next day, the patients ask the exact same questions I answered the day before.

I can relate to this easily. My sister, who works in tech, can patiently explain something about computers to me, and I can genuinely listen, try to understand, and still end up no further ahead. (And despite all these conversations, I cannot even call to mind a specific thing about computers that she has explained.)

It can take a long time to understand an explanation when you have no prior knowledge to provide scaffolding. Sometimes, no matter how well explained, it takes a long time to process an answer that isn't what you hoped to hear. I had a surgical patient who came in a few times with a bowel obstruction. He had a history of surgeries in his abdomen, which is the commonest reason for bowel obstructions. Normally, the organs have slippery surfaces and can slide over each other within the abdomen, but surgery can cause the organs to stick together with scar tissue called 'adhesions'. When a bowel is twisted up with adhesions it's hard for things to get through, and the contents of the bowel (not only what you've had to eat and drink, but also the many litres of fluid your intestines pump out daily to help with digestion) back up and spill out the top end through vomiting.

He was exhausted from multiple hospital admissions in only a few months, and desperate to fix this problem once and for all. He couldn't understand why the surgeons wouldn't just 'do something' to fix it. We talked many times about the fact that the problem had been caused by operations he had needed in the past, and that we wanted to avoid operating again if possible because it would cause more adhesions. I explained it in as many ways as I knew how. Even so, every morning on the ward round, he would say the same thing.

'No offence to the quality of the food here, but it doesn't exactly have a Michelin star. I can't keep coming back here, you've got to do something. It's not fair on me and it's not fair on the staff.'

Most days after ward rounds he would ask the nurse the same questions again, and the nurse would call me. I would do my best to answer his questions, while in the back of my mind my to-do list flashed bright red.

He would repeat his Michelin-star line each time, and I would do my part and chuckle.

It went on like this for nearly a week, until one day he added, 'I can't keep calling ambulances every few weeks,' his voice cracking a tiny bit as he said it.

It should have happened sooner, but it was then I realised I had to let go of wanting to move on to the next task. I needed to take some time to actually listen. I moved a chair beside his bed and sat down.

He told me he lived alone, and although he had friends and family nearby, he didn't want to be a burden on them, so he handled his health problems on his own. In the space of a year he had come to hospital maybe six times for serious and life-threatening problems. He didn't want to trouble people to give him a ride, so every time he fell ill he had to call an ambulance. Writing this, it occurs to me that an ambulance costs about a hundred dollars each time, although he never mentioned the cost and I didn't ask. I had known about all these hospital visits, could have rattled off his medical history without a second thought, but it was the first time I had really stopped to think what the past year must have been like for him.

We are taught in medical school, and as human beings we know instinctively, I think, how therapeutic it can be for patients to just let them talk. But working comes with different priorities. Perhaps we are hoping to leave on time for once. Perhaps we have had three phone calls from another patient's nurse to remind us they are waiting for discharge papers.

For days I had been hearing this patient say 'I can't keep doing this' and understood it as a demand for surgery, a treatment which I believed would cause more harm than good. But I think what he was really asking for was for someone to recognise how much he had been through. I think we were the only people he didn't feel he had to be strong for.

'You've had a hell of a year,' I said gently. 'You must be exhausted.'

Tears welled up in his eyes and I handed him a tissue. We kept talking for a long while, and for the first time since I met him I didn't try to explain or communicate my point of view.

'So you can't do an operation to fix me,' he said gruffly. 'When will this happen again?'

Vital Signs

The truth was, I didn't know, and I told him so. It might be in a week or it might never happen again.

He sighed. 'I guess I better go home then. No offence to the quality of the food here, but it doesn't exactly have a Michelin star.'

He winked at me, and this time my chuckle was genuine.

CHAPTER 17:

Long stayers

MOST PEOPLE COME to the hospital and stay for a few days, or perhaps a week. Then there are the long stayers. Their situations vary. There is the patient who is on your list for the entire three months of a rotation. The patient who has become part of the furniture. The long, slow recovery from a difficult and complicated surgery. The long, slow decline over months in the ICU before it becomes clear that even with our best efforts, this person isn't going to survive. The chronic illness that brings someone back every few weeks. The person whose health has recovered, but who doesn't have anywhere to go and so cannot be safely discharged. The person whose discharge summary with the long list of problems and interventions they have had in hospital was 'prepped' by the house officers who did this job before you, and will be left 'prepped' for the next person when you leave.

Every rotation I've had as a doctor has had at least one of these, and every doctor I know has a list of long stayers they've cared for. Long stayers get to know us over months of brief conversations. They banter, give us shit on the ward rounds, and tell our bosses we made messy work of putting in their IV line. We book scans for them every week, and commiserate with them when this week's scan result is no better than the last. Every junior doctor in the hospital has heard of them, either in a handover meeting or because they had been called on a long day by a nurse who was concerned about them. Long stayers become legends. We have had patients who have been in hospital for over a year.

Being in hospital for months is my nightmare. The food is average, and so is the WiFi. Staying that long, a hospital-acquired infection is virtually inevitable. You'll be covered in bruises from blood tests and IV lines. IV lines tend to fail within a few days, and have to be changed to prevent infection anyway. If you started with good veins, the house officers who are called to get an IV line in will start to find it more and more difficult, which means more and more painful needle jabs. A hospital long stayer ends up with no usable veins, and will often need a special long-term IV line called a PICC line.

At some point you will become a medical emergency. The doctors will be so worried that they'll call your family in, so worried that they consult with the ICU. Maybe you'll have to go there. After that, the trauma of being so ill that a code team rushed to your bedside will flash back whenever you hear the ward's emergency bell.

Being there for a long time doesn't mean you'll be in a single room — instead, there will be a revolving door of patients wheeled into and out of your four-bed room. Some of them will be wonderful, and you'll become lifelong friends. Others will be made grumpy and miserable by what brought them into hospital. Or, you will be the grumpy and miserable one, and they will be so chirpy and annoying that you'll want to strangle them. Some will snore, or get sick overnight so that the flurry of nurses and doctors will make it impossible to get any sleep. Some will die, right there behind a curtain just across the room.

You'll lose muscle tone from being in a hospital bed all day. You'll lose weight from feeling too sick to eat. Your body won't look or feel like your own, and some days you will just wear the hospital gown because you don't have the energy to put on clothes. Most of the staff will be kind, and you'll come to see them almost like family. Some will be rough or rude or just too busy to treat you like anything more than a job on their long to-do list. The sound of call bells will become background noise to your life, until you learn to tune it out. You'll wonder if the nurses are tuning it out when you push yours and wait and wait.

If you weren't depressed before, you probably are now. When people come to visit you, they are rewarded with expensive parking and constant interruptions by staff coming to talk to you, taking your blood pressure or temperature, giving you medications, asking your lunch order and emptying your rubbish bin. People have lives of their own, and over time the visits will grow less and less frequent.

I will carry my little collection of long stayers with me forever.

Sharon had cancer, and she was going to die from it. It was the kind of cancer we can't do very much for, but there were some palliative options. She had fasted day after day for procedures that would help ease her symptoms, not able to eat until she was either back from the procedure or (more commonly) bumped off the list at four in the afternoon. We would sometimes take her an Anzac biscuit, her favourite, as a treat on days she was allowed to eat.

She was living alone and finding it harder and harder to manage, but she was fiercely independent and didn't want to be in a rest home.

Paul had spent weeks in the ICU before he was well enough

to come to the ward. For a while, I thought for sure that he was going to die, but he turned a corner. He teased me whenever I dropped my pen and paper on ward rounds (which seemed to happen every day).

Iokua gave us a huge smile every time he saw us, and finished the ward round with a fist bump for every single member of the team.

Danny was an alcoholic, and drinking too much had given him pancreatitis. He had started drinking to cope with a traumatic childhood, and every night he had downed as many beers as he could afford. In hospital his pancreatitis improved, but his drinking had also made him homeless and he didn't have anywhere safe to go. We knew he would probably return to drinking when he left the hospital, and we told him that was a bad idea, but it wasn't a reason to keep him once his medical problems settled.

Fred's wife, Mary, had gone home and broken her hip right after visiting him in hospital, where he was staying because he'd broken his. We put them in the same room, until it got too confusing having Mr and Mrs with the same last name in the same room and the orderly took Mary's notes to Fred's scan by mistake. The two of them celebrated their wedding anniversary in the hospital with their loved ones gathered around.

Angela had a torn oesophagus, which healed slowly over months of not being allowed to eat or drink, all nutrition given into a vein.

Ikenasio had cognitive impairment, which meant that he couldn't remember to use the call bell, and would shout 'Nurse!' at the top of his lungs whenever he needed something. He would also say 'Thank you, Nurse' every morning to my registrar.

Kevin, a Chinese man in hospital with heart problems, explained on the ward round that his wife was at home and had bad arthritis, so they were 'two people, three legs'. One morning we had a relieving registrar who spoke Mandarin. I had told him about Kevin and his wife in advance. 'He says he has limited English, but that was a better joke than I could have made in Mandarin,' I said. When the registrar met Kevin, they spoke in Mandarin for a long while. At one point, the registrar chuckled, and interpreted for me. 'Two people, three legs.'

Hone called Gaby 'Bub', and wanted to move north to spend his last few weeks or months closer to his tūrangawaewae. He had lung cancer, the kind you get from smoking, the kind that disproportionately affects Māori. I don't think he saw the point of staying in hospital if we couldn't cure him, and he once gestured accusingly at our (admittedly handsome) registrar, and said, 'Let me out of here, I'm sick of looking at his bloody beautiful face.'

Vea had been transferred from her home on a Pacific island with a mysterious infection that was easily diagnosed with advanced testing that her local hospital did not have. She was with us on antibiotics for many weeks, and her devoted children took shifts at her bedside, reading her the Bible and giving traditional healing massages.

We learned greetings in their languages to use on the ward rounds. We got to know their families and saw photos of their pets. We heard their stories, and began to understand how they had become ill. We heard about the horrific murder they witnessed as a young person, which had driven them to drink; about how everyone in their family had smoked so they had started smoking; about how they hadn't taken the antibiotics we prescribed last time because they didn't have five dollars for the prescription fee. We tried to discharge them and found they were planning to return to living in a garage, or a caravan with steps they could barely climb.

We saw them more than we saw our own families. When they got good news, we celebrated with them. When the news was bad, our hearts sank. I wept buckets when I got the news that Sharon had died.

CHAPTER 13:

Death

AT MEDICAL SCHOOL we learn, in detail that feels excruciating and yet only scratches the surface, the processes that happen at a cell, organ and whole-body level to keep our bodies alive without us even needing to think about it. Most of these body processes rely in some way on oxygen. It is essential for turning the food we eat into fuel our cells can use. Staying alive from one minute to the next requires our bodies to do two things: to move air in and out of the lungs to fill our blood with oxygen; and to move that oxygen-rich blood from the lungs to the heart, and from the heart to the rest of the body.

If either one of these processes stops, we call it an 'arrest'. In an arrest, our job becomes simple. Keep air moving in and out. Keep blood moving around — most importantly to the brain, which can't survive for long without oxygen. Find out whether the person's heart needs an electric shock, and if it does, give it one. Try to figure out why they have arrested, and fix that underlying cause if possible.

Vital Signs

We rehearse this process over and over in resuscitation training and in simulations until it is nearly automatic. Compressing
the chest to squeeze the heart from the outside and move
the blood through. Opening the airway and ventilating the
lungs so that the blood will have oxygen. Delivering an electric
shock to stun the heart out of an abnormal rhythm and allow
it to resume the normal 'sinus' rhythm, set by pacemaker cells
in the heart that allow it to beat without being told. I have
given cardiopulmonary resuscitation (CPR) to a resuscitation
dummy on perhaps 50 occasions since the beginning of
medical school. I have given CPR to a person once.

One evening I was holding the house officer 'resus pager'.
It went off, the text message indicating there was a cardiac
arrest on Ward 6. I was at the other end of the hospital, and
resuscitation attempts were already well underway when I
arrived. The patient had been found unresponsive by his nurse,
and the resuscitation team, four more senior doctors and a
handful of other house officers were already there managing
his airway and looking through his notes, trying to figure out
why he had arrested.

I joined the queue of junior doctors and ward nurses who
were taking turns at performing chest compressions. This is a
physically exhausting task, and taking it in turns prevents us
from getting so tired we don't compress the chest effectively.

When it was my turn, I knelt up on the hospital bed with
my hands over his mid-sternum, and my muscle memory took
over. One third the depth of the chest, 100–120 compressions
per minute. He must have been bleeding into his lungs, and
with every compression more blood was forced out into his
mouth and then down his chin. I looked away. My only job was
to keep blood moving from his heart to his brain.

We got him back for a little while, only to lose him again.
This happened three more times. When after the third arrest
we could not get his heart and lungs to work on their own

— what we call return of spontaneous circulation (ROSC) — the senior doctors talked among themselves, and agreed that we had done everything we could. They asked the whole team if anyone had concerns about stopping our efforts at resuscitation. Nobody did. We stopped compressions, and removed the bag and tube we had been using to breathe for him. The nurses cleaned up the room, which was littered with the equipment we had used in our efforts to save him, and changed the bloodied sheets. They cleaned the blood from his face and covered him with a clean blanket, ready for his family to arrive.

Afterwards, we sat down as a team to debrief the resuscitation. Medically speaking, it had been textbook. We had worked seamlessly as a team, the senior doctors had provided good leadership and had done all the right things to look for reversible causes of his collapse. He had received gold-standard care from the moment he was found unconscious by his nurse until the moment we stopped CPR. It helped me to hear that. It helped to sit for a minute, acknowledging what had just happened. Then it was on with the rest of the shift. A patient had oral thrush and needed an antifungal, someone else had a rash, and about ten people needed laxatives. It wasn't until the drive home that I let myself cry.

I still remember my first-ever patient death. I remember her name, and can easily recall her face in my mind. I was a fourth-year medical student, brand new to the clinical years of medical school and a week or two into my first rotation. She was in her eighties, and had come in only a few days before I joined the team, brought in because her family were worried about her nausea and the yellow tinge to her eyes and skin. She had lost 10 kg in weight over the last few months. In medical school we memorise the classical presentations of illnesses, and any medical student can tell you that painless jaundice with weight loss means pancreatic cancer. Her CT scan confirmed the worst: a big tumour at the head of the pancreas that was compressing her bile duct and part of her small intestine.

It was too advanced to operate. Even if her cancer had been amenable to an operation, she wouldn't have survived the surgery. The multidisciplinary meeting (MDM), where the surgeons, oncologists and pathologists meet to make a treatment plan for cancer patients, had agreed that even palliative chemotherapy wouldn't be in her best interests. It was decided that the most suitable option was to offer what we call 'best supportive care' to manage her symptoms and allow her to enjoy whatever time she had left.

In the end, that time was short. The cancer obstructed her small bowel, meaning that no food could pass through. She didn't want a stent or a feeding tube. She just wanted to die. One morning on the ward round she begged my registrar to end her life. The registrar said that the government was deciding if that would be an option in the future (this would have been when the End of Life Choice Bill was before Parliament). It struck me at the time as an odd thing to say; it seemed clear to me, with all my two weeks' experience in clinical medicine, that this woman wouldn't live to see that Bill enacted into law. Thinking about it now, I have a bit more empathy for the position the registrar had been put in. She was in her third year as a doctor, and had only been a registrar for a couple of months. I have no idea what I would have said if a patient had asked that of me.

The patient passed quickly but seemed to suffer greatly. Her skin was the colour of butter and the jaundice gave her an unbearable itch. Her children and grandchildren visited often, spooned ice chips into her dry mouth and read to her from the books of poetry on her bedside table. Then one morning she was gone from our patient list. She had died overnight. I was sad, but also glad for her.

Later that year, sad over the unexpected death of another

patient, I remember asking a medical registrar I really admired whether the deaths keep affecting you the same way after years of doing the job. 'No,' she said simply. 'You see so many. It's not that you stop caring, but you can't feel sad all the time.'

I remember thinking that wouldn't be true for me. I am a sensitive soul, moved to tears by virtually any strong emotion, and I care deeply about other people. Surely the end of a human life couldn't leave me unmoved, no matter how many I saw. And yet, after only a year in the job, I see what she means. It's still sad when a patient dies, especially when it's a patient who has been under my care for a while, but I don't cry in the bathroom every time.

When a person dies, a doctor has to pronounce them dead. We are not taught how to do this in medical school, at least not formally. In the final year of study a particularly keen student with particularly keen teachers might have had the opportunity to observe a couple of patients being pronounced dead. A house officer might have informally talked to us about the death certificate process. But, like many parts of the job, we learn this strange new responsibility by doing.

People who die at home are usually pronounced dead by their GP, who might see the body some hours later, when there is little question that they are deceased. In hospital, where the death has usually occurred only minutes ago, up to perhaps an hour, this involves a physical examination for the absence of signs of life.

To pronounce a person dead I must observe for a full minute that they are not breathing, while feeling for a full minute that there is no pulse. I can get away with using my phone to tell the time for most other things, but for this task it feels disrespectful, so I have a nursing fob watch with a second hand which I use only for this purpose. Next, I place a stethoscope on the chest to confirm the absence of heart sounds. Finally, I open the patient's eyes and shine a pupil torch (another tool my phone can replace in all other contexts) to confirm that the pupils are fixed and dilated. At two in the morning on a dark hospital ward, this examination often feels more spiritual than medical.

Sometimes the patient's family is at the bedside. This is easier when the patient is someone I have looked after personally, so I've met the family, and can at least guess the shape of their grief so that I can tread lightly around it. After hours, it helps if the nurse is someone who has looked after the person and knows the family. Sometimes I have nothing to go on except the clinical notes. What I am looking for is: was this death expected? What is the likely cause of the death, and how did we try to treat the condition? Did the family agree with the plan for the patient's care, or did they have concerns? At best, I am hoping to make the ritual of pronouncing them dead a useful part of the process of mourning. If nothing else, I am hoping to avoid adding to their trauma.

'My name is Izzy and I'm one of the doctors. I'm so sorry for your loss. To confirm that your mum has died, I need to perform a physical examination. Would it be okay if I do that now, or do you need some more time?'

I am always prepared for the family to say they need more time, but they never do. Some murmur about getting it over with, while others, even in their grief, are conscious of not making me wait. I think for some families it can help a little bit to have the certainty of a doctor telling them that, yes indeed, their loved one has died.

It isn't always easy for families to tell. Sometimes the noise of an anti-pressure air mattress can be mistaken for breathing. Sometimes the person has died while they have 'high flow' running — a kind of respiratory support where warmed, humidified air is pushed quickly into the nostrils to help support breathing and keep the airways open. Sometimes people's eyes play tricks on them.

I had a patient who died in my first month as a doctor. He had come in with a heart attack and we gave what we call a 'guarded prognosis' — we warned his family that although we would give him the best care available, we expected that he might not survive. He was an older Pasifika man, with a beautiful family who crowded into the awkward little room in the Emergency Department. I had actually just gone in to check on him as he took his final breaths. His children crowded around him and wept openly, with one of his daughters rocking against the railing and saying 'Dad, no' again and again. When it was time to examine him, his granddaughter told me that she had seen him moving, and asked if I was sure. I gently explained that the movement of his family around him was shifting the bed, causing his body to shift slightly. He was gone.

After the physical examination, there is paperwork. My hospital is unique in having a 24-hour Bereavement Care service. Its staff attend every death in the hospital. They explain to families the next steps: taking the patient's body to the hospital mortuary and arranging for collection by a funeral director. They also explain to clueless young doctors like me how to complete the paperwork.

These days, death certificates are completed electronically through an online portal called 'Death Docs'. Once I've figured out my RealMe login, sworn at the default browser, quit that browser and opened Chrome, and logged back into my RealMe, the certificate itself is fairly simple. I state the person's name, National Health Index (NHI) number, date of birth, date and place of death, and the direct and antecedent causes of death. The direct cause of death is the final step in the chain of events that led to the person dying — for example, sepsis. Antecedent causes are the steps further back in that chain of events — for example, the sepsis might have been caused by cellulitis. Going back further, the cellulitis might have been caused by a diabetic ulcer giving bacteria a way through the skin. This information is used by the Ministry of Health to compile statistics about causes of death in New Zealand.

I confirm that the death does not need to be reported to the coroner, which it might be if it is unexplained, if it happened because of a medical procedure, or if the patient was a person in state care such as a psychiatric institution or a prison. I complete a cremation certificate confirming there is no reason it would be desirable not to proceed for cremation. This involves checking that there is no cardiac pacemaker or other implanted device that might explode in the furnace. I am also asked to certify that I personally attended to the patient in their final illness, stating when I last saw them alive and how soon after death I examined the body, and what steps I took to satisfy myself that they had died.

This section of the cremation certificate has given rise to the slightly morbid practice among junior doctors of 'sighting' patients who are expected to die. If a team's patient is dying, and might pass away after hours, we put a task on our electronic Task Manager reminding us to 'sight' the patient — to lay eyes on them, partly to check if they are comfortable, but mostly so that the on-call doctor has seen them alive and can complete death paperwork if necessary.

Once, on what had already been a fairly horrible on-call shift, I went to sight a patient who had been receiving end-of-life palliative care. His family were all in the room crying, which should have given me pause, but it didn't.

'Kia ora, my name is Izzy and I'm one of the doctors. I've just come to check in on your dad.'

The family stared at me. Slowly, I approached the bed. It became very clear that the patient was pale and not breathing.

'Oh, do you think he might have passed away?' I said softly.

'Yes. A couple of hours ago,' said a grandson, and I was left to murmur my regret at their sad loss, and make a hasty and mortified retreat from the room. Since then, I always check with the nurses before attempting to sight someone.

The alternative to sighting is that the usual team completes the paperwork the next day. In some ways this is preferable — the team who took care of the patient is better placed to give an accurate account of the cause of death. But it can be traumatising for families to have to wait to pick up their loved one's body until the doctors can complete the paperwork.

The first time I completed a death certificate for a patient whose death had been pronounced by another doctor after hours, I did it all wrong. It was 8.30 a.m. on the busiest day of my week and we were on our ward round when I got a call from Bereavement Care to say that the paperwork needed to be done because the funeral director was arriving at 9 a.m. It was the first I'd heard that the patient had died, as it hadn't been handed over, and I hadn't yet noticed that there was someone missing from my long patient list. All deaths are sad, but this one especially so — she had been in her sixties and had suffered a huge bleed into her brain. Her husband hadn't left her side in the three days she was with us before she passed away.

I went to the ward to meet the Bereavement Care staff and complete the paperwork, only to find that the body had already been taken to the mortuary at the other end of the hospital some hours earlier. The person from Bereavement Care offered to meet me on the ward and I completed the cremation certificate, stating that I had not seen the body after death, and that she had been examined by the on-call house officer.

The next day I was on leave when I got a call from the manager of Bereavement Care. The cremation certificate had been declined — I hadn't realised I needed to see the person's body myself in order to complete the paperwork. The family had been planning to have her cremated that day and were understandably distraught. To complicate matters, Auckland was in lockdown and I couldn't visit the funeral home to

Vital Signs

examine her. We managed to arrange for it to be done by video conference. I scrambled to tidy my unwashed hair, and threw a semi-respectable shirt over my pyjamas. Then from the tidiest part of my room I made a solemn FaceTime call to the funeral director. He showed me my patient in her casket, the mortuary make-up making her look almost as though she was sleeping. 'She looks peaceful,' I murmured. I thanked him awkwardly and logged in to amend the certificate.

CHAPTER 19:

Non-adherence

PEOPLE COME TO us with a problem. We ask questions, perform an examination, run tests and come to a diagnosis. We recommend a course of treatment. The patient then decides whether or not to do what we say.

Not all prescriptions we write will be collected, and not all medications collected will be taken. If they are taken, it may not be regularly. Most people will fail to take their prescribed medications at least some of the time. We call this 'non-adherence'.

There are lots of reasons for non-adherence. People might not be able to collect a prescription because they can't afford the five-dollar prescription fee, or don't have transport to get to a pharmacy where prescriptions are free. They might not have time to collect their prescription. They might have read about the risks of a medication and decided they don't want to take it, or they might have tried the medication and been put off by side effects. The problem they went to the doctor with might feel better, meaning they don't feel like they need treatment.

They might remember to take the medication some times, but not others. I definitely don't have perfect adherence when I am on regular medication. I have forgotten doses for days at a time, or forgotten that I've taken a dose and accidentally doubled up.

The type of non-adherence I struggle with the most is when patients leave hospital against medical advice. In a perfect society where people had every advantage and opportunity available to them their whole lives, and where the health system treated everyone equally well, it would be easier for me to accept when people choose to self-discharge. As it stands, people face discrimination and poor treatment in our health system because of their ethnicity, social class or stereotypes about their health conditions. People's lives are also hard and complicated, and the choice to stay and get the care they need isn't equally available to all our patients.

If you are in precarious employment with no sick days, and have no savings to fall back on, staying in hospital to receive care might mean your rent goes unpaid or your kids don't eat. If there is nobody else to look after your husband with dementia, staying in hospital might mean he sets the house on fire trying to make himself dinner. If an addiction controls your life, staying in hospital means losing access to that substance until you are discharged. Being a doctor has taught me what a privilege it is to be able to put your own health first.

When someone tells the nurses they are planning to leave the hospital against medical advice, a nurse will try to convince them to stay, and calls the house officer. The house officer talks to them to understand why they are planning to leave, and also tries to convince them to stay. We tell them that it is their right to leave, but we think it would be a mistake. We explain why we think it's a good idea for them to be in hospital, and what we are worried might happen if they leave.

If they are still insistent on going, we ask them to sign a form acknowledging that these risks have been explained to them. Worsening infection, sepsis, death. Recurrent upper gastrointestinal bleeding, hypovolaemic shock, death. Cardiac arrhythmia, cardiac arrest, death.

Patients are usually happy to sign the form accepting these risks. They know their lives better than we do, and their reason for leaving means more to them than our worst-case scenarios.

In that case, we do everything we can to make their discharge safe. If they won't stay in hospital for IV antibiotics, we try to at least get them a prescription for tablets. If they won't stay because they are planning to leave Auckland, we call the hospital where they are going to see if we can arrange a transfer. If they won't stay for the colonoscopy we're concerned will show cancer, we organise one as an outpatient. We try to avoid referring the person back to their GP if we can. It costs money to go to a GP, and a lot of our patients have put off seeking help because they don't have the money, transport or time off work to get there.

They leave, and we worry. One of my patients left against medical advice with an upper gastrointestinal bleed. Every day for a week he had told us he was sick of being in hospital, and every day we told him we didn't think he was safe to leave. A gastroscopy hadn't managed to identify a source of bleeding, but his blood count was still dropping. The next step would be a 'pill cam', where a camera the size of a large pill is swallowed and travels through the intestines, recording the whole way. These were in short supply, and it would be another few days before we could give him one.

Vital Signs

For a few days I managed to convince him to stay, but one evening when I was on call the nurses told me he had decided he really was going to leave. My best efforts to convince him one more time failed. I asked him to at least let me organise a follow-up blood test the next week, to check that he wasn't still bleeding out.

He didn't have transport and lived alone, so I requested a home visit from the phlebotomy service. The following week I got a notification that he hadn't been home when they called, and they hadn't been able to reach him. I tried calling, but his phone went straight to voicemail. I left a message, asking in a tone as light as I could manage whether he would like me to reschedule his appointment. I called his GP to see if they had any other phone numbers I could try, but they didn't even have his current address.

I tried to call a few more times over the following week but never managed to get through. I tried not to imagine him dead on the floor in a pool of bloody vomit. I briefly considered going to his house to check he was okay, but knew that would be a violation of boundaries.

Months later, when I was on another run entirely, I saw him. He was in hospital for a completely different reason, in the same room as a patient my team was looking after. When he saw me he waved and gave me a big grin. 'Hey Doc,' he said in a cheeky tone, 'I finally got that blood test.'

'Glad to hear it,' I said, grinning back.

CHAPTER 20:

Taking the wheel

I WAS 27 when I learned to drive a car. I left home right around the age when most people learn, and didn't have anyone to teach me, and as an environmentalist I didn't want to rely on a car for transport. I took the bus or walked. When I was twenty, while I was home for Christmas, Mum decided to teach me to drive, so I got a learner's licence. Within twenty seconds of my first practical driving lesson starting, I had managed to crash Mum's quite new car into a stack of pallets, and that was the end of that.

In my fourth year of medical school I realised that I really wanted to do my fifth year at a rural hospital. The rural programme requires you to have a licence and your own car, for obvious reasons. There is no public transport in small-town

Vital Signs

New Zealand. So I went on the AA website and signed up to do driving lessons with Ernie.

Ernie was a gentle and softly spoken man, with a dual-controlled car that he could brake independently if need be. For my first lesson, he drove us to a big empty car park in St Kilda and I practised doing figure of eights until I got a feel for the steering wheel. He stayed calm as I made jerky work of figuring out the brakes. I was shaking for the whole lesson, and when he switched back into the driver's seat I was so relieved.

The next week he drove me to St Kilda again and I did my figure of eights. At the end of the lesson he told me I was going to drive us back into town. I was so nervous I nearly tossed my cookies, but Ernie told me that it was okay, and that I was going to be a good, safe driver. I survived turning left at a roundabout, then driving the straight arterial route into town. Like most new drivers, I hugged the kerb, and Ernie said calmly, 'Out to you!' until I was correctly positioned in the lane. I just about mounted the footpath taking a corner that wasn't 90 degrees. Ernie calmly applied his brake pedal and talked me through correcting my mistake.

Over the course of fifteen lessons, Ernie turned me from someone who hadn't ever been behind the wheel into someone capable of passing her restricted licence test. During most of our lessons I would verbalise the anxiety and dread I felt at doing something wrong. He would always tell me in response, 'You have to tell yourself you're going to be a good, safe driver.'

I guess it cost about a thousand dollars all up to learn to drive, and it was the best thousand dollars I've ever spent. I remember thinking at the time what a stark contrast there was between driving school, where I was taught a difficult new set of skills with patience and compassion, and medical school, where I was expected to know skills that I had never had the opportunity to learn.

Our teachers in clinical medicine are not always professional teachers. They are the mum-and-dad driving instructors of the world, grasping the passenger handle and drawing sharp intakes of breath at every corner. Some even snap at us for small mistakes and laugh at us when we don't have knowledge that seem obvious to them. In medicine I have met a few Ernies, with calm voices that guided me through new skills and gently corrected me when necessary, but it is not the norm.

Medical-school training in New Zealand lasts six years. Half of that time is spent at university, sitting in lectures and tutorials, learning the names of the muscles, bones, nerves and blood vessels, the way medications work, and how the body's normal processes are disrupted in different disease states. The other half is spent in hospitals: the start of the decade or so we will spend as apprentices learning to care for the sick. During that time we learn to take a history from patients, how to perform a physical examination, how to order and interpret blood tests and X-rays, and how to perform and read ECGs. Those three years of clinical medicine give us, we hope, the knowledge and skills that we'll need to be a new doctor. They also teach us how to *be* as a doctor.

This is called the hidden curriculum, or 'medical socialisation', and was the hardest part of medical school for me. I loved meeting patients and I was interested in learning everything I could about different diseases and treatments, but I struggled to adjust to the hospital culture. The things I had to navigate were legion: how to banter lightly with the people whose opinions and feedback decided my entire grade. Who was called Dr, who was Mr, Mrs, Ms or Prof, and who just used their first name. When it was appropriate to ask questions and when I should be seen and not heard. How to be eager but unobtrusive, dedicated but not annoying. How to balance the expectation of the medical school that we should be at the hospital all day with the obvious wish of the staff that we would just go home and let them get some work done in peace.

Vital Signs

How to understand medical speak — not just the jargon we use for disease names and drugs but the ordinary words that have different meanings in a hospital. In a clinic, a consultant once told me to go to interview a patient. 'Mrs Anders is in Room 3, go and get her story.' I went to talk to her. She had cancer, and she shared with me the story of her diagnosis, the treatments she had tried so far, and how lately it had mostly been bad news. I squeezed her hand and told her sincerely how sorry I was that it was happening. The consultant was perplexed when I went to report back to him. 'But did you ask her what symptoms she's having at the moment?'

In medicine, it transpired, someone's 'story' doesn't really mean their story. It's just a quirky way to refer to taking a history of their symptoms.

The first feedback session I had from a consultant in medical school was tough. He told me that I was keen, had good knowledge and asked good questions, but that the registrars didn't like me. He didn't really say why, and wasn't specific enough to make it useful feedback in terms of changing my approach.

I hated coming to the hospital after that. I felt exposed and vulnerable, worried that I would see one of the doctors I had admired and regarded as a mentor without realising they couldn't stand me. I had a few more bad experiences, and decided in desperation that I needed to leave the city I had chosen to train in. I applied to do a rural immersion year away from the rest of my cohort, and I was accepted. I spent a full year living with two boys I'd barely spoken to before. We became good friends, all studying at the same small hospital and signing up for whatever clinics and surgeries we wanted to see each week.

Years of therapy later, I can recognise what that feedback I was given in medical school uncovered in me: a desperation to be liked, and a fear that I am fundamentally unlikeable. I have done enough work on liking myself now that it stings a little less. Sometimes I think clinical medicine is a circle of hell designed specifically for smart, anxious, competitive people who want to be liked. One classmate, who was earnest and well meaning and sometimes soothed her anxiety by being a little bit too talkative, was told in as many words that she needed to change her personality, because nobody wanted a doctor like her.

As students, we would rotate to a new team every four weeks or so. I have always made a terrible first impression, and it was exhausting to be constantly trying to impress a new group of people whose opinion of me determined my grades. I would come home at the end of every day exhausted from trying not to seem like a weirdo or a fool. I would anxiously blurt out stupid things, and then replay them in my head each night.

Our place in the hospital hierarchy sat somewhere below the cockroaches, but above the fleas. The meaner nurses would openly bully us, taking out the frustrations of their jobs and relationships with doctors on us because they knew that nobody would stop them. The house officers were mostly kind, I guess because they remembered what it was like to be in our shoes. The registrars gave us the most direct teaching, and the quality of your learning experience was largely determined by the quality of your registrars.

Medical socialisation involves learning our profession's jargon, especially the terms you won't find in a textbook. One of my classmates lost sight of a fast-moving surgical ward round after the registrar said that Mrs Brown was the next patient to see. He searched the ward for a patient called Mrs Brown, but there was nobody with that name. Eventually he asked one of the house officers, who chuckled and explained that seeing Mrs Brown meant going downstairs to get coffee.

For a science-adjacent profession, doctors are a superstitious bunch. We don't say 'the Q word'. I learned this rule as a fifth-year student at a small-town Emergency Department. A patient asked how my day was going, and I told her it was pretty quiet.

'Ooh, Izzy, now you've gone and done it,' said one of the nurses.

Within fifteen minutes, two critically injured people had arrived by ambulance, requiring an emergency call-out to the whole of the small hospital to summon the senior staff to assist in their care. I didn't say the Q word after that, just in case. My other superstition is that I always take enough equipment for a second try at putting in an IV line, because some part of me believes that if I am humble, the cannulation gods will look favourably on me and I will get it on the first try.

Medical socialisation is also learning to survive in an environment where burnt-out staff are sometimes openly dismissive of patients and colleagues, and where you have to give stressed people some latitude for their rudeness. It's about learning to pick your battles and bitching to your colleagues about it later.

For women, it is learning to respond with grace when you are constantly mistaken for a nurse. This happens even when the nurses wear uniforms that say 'nurse' and doctors are in plain clothes, or when 'doctor' is embroidered on our scrubs. It happens when we introduce ourselves as doctors.

This is a tricky problem to describe, because in complaining about it, I need to be clear that nurses are probably the most important workforce in the hospital, and the hospital would grind to a halt without them long before it would without me. Many nurses have a wealth of expertise from decades working in their field, and may know what to do when I don't. But I am not a nurse. I am a doctor. I went to university for six years to become a doctor, and 60 per cent of the doctors who graduated in my cohort were women. In fact, for decades the majority of medical graduates have been women, and yet if I say to someone I am meeting casually that I work in a hospital, they will assume I work as a nurse.

This stereotype means that patients whose doctors have faithfully seen them on rounds will leave the hospital after a week and complain that they never once saw a doctor. Māori and Pasifika colleagues get a double dose of bias, and sometimes even get mistaken for healthcare assistants or cleaners.

One of the learned behaviours I find most frustrating in myself and other people in medicine is professional defensiveness. If a patient (or even another doctor) describes a situation where a doctor has been accused of doing or saying something ill-advised or wrong, especially if it is reported in the media, other doctors will rush to defend their colleague. 'We don't know all the facts,' they will say. 'We have only heard one side of the story.'

While this is possibly true, it is indicative of a tendency in doctors to believe another doctor's word over a patient's. The problem with this is that the doctor–patient relationship is one in which the doctor wields immense power and can do immense harm. This is even more true when the patient is structurally disadvantaged in society because of their ethnicity, class, disability, gender or sexuality. When we defend an unnamed doctor because they have a hard job, we ignore the much harder job of the patient: to suffer whatever symptoms they are having, and at the same time navigate a healthcare system that can be confusing, impenetrable and sometimes outright discriminatory and hostile.

I have long been interested in the struggles of women with chronic illness, chronic pain or medically unexplained symptoms, yet some days I notice I am internally rolling my eyes at someone who is desperate and frustrated that I cannot give her an answer or take her pain away. Some days I hear myself casually saying that a patient is 'paining' when running through who might be discharged today and who likely won't.

Vital Signs

It is a constant battle to resist internalising and reproducing the discrimination I was so determined to challenge when I first came into medicine.

I want to be one of the good ones. I've learned that everyone thinks they're one of the good ones, including doctors I've overheard being openly racist or sexist, or the ones who say all the right things about social justice but bully and belittle their juniors.

Historically, medical students were mostly from demographics that are structurally advantaged: wealthy, Pākehā, from high-decile or private schools. This is changing as a result of affirmative-action policies that give priority to Māori and Pasifika, low socioeconomic status and former refugee students who want to study to be doctors. Predictably, these policies have been met with some resistance by those who had become accustomed to having an advantage. How unfair that all of a sudden these policies have levelled the playing field.

On the first day of medical school, Professor Peter Crampton (our dean at the time and one of the architects of Otago University's Mirror on Society selection policy, which gives priority to students from disadvantaged groups) welcomed us to the medical profession. He told us that although 59 per cent of us were women, only 1 per cent of us had attended low-decile schools, and that for the first time in medical school history, Māori and Pasifika students were represented in our cohort at population levels.

It will be decades before the playing field is truly level, and patients can find doctors who look like them at all levels of the medical profession. Patients need this, but students need it too. We need to have role models in medicine who look like us and share some of the same life experiences. Most of all, we need role models who will be gentle when we mount the kerb, and who will remind us: 'You have to tell yourself you're going to be a good, safe doctor.'

CHAPTER 21:

Goodnight moon

SIX MONTHS INTO being a doctor (or three months if your first rotation was Gen Med) you become eligible to do night shifts.

On most rosters, nights come in sets of three or four, followed by three days off to sleep and recover.

The daytime before the first night shift feels like a day off. It is a day for errands, laundry, long walks and flat whites. Some people can sleep during the day before night shifts, but I have never been able to manage more than perhaps an hour-long nap. I eat a light dinner (anything heavy will make me sleepy) and drink a plunger of black coffee.

Around 8 p.m. the dread sets in. Stress hormones course through me, making my stomach churn (or perhaps that's the coffee). At 9 p.m. I get in my little Toyota Yaris. I stop at the Wild Bean cafe, the only place in the neighbourhood open that late, to get my hazelnut latte.

I arrive at the hospital by 9.30 p.m, change into scrubs and make my way to get a handover from the long-day doctor. I was late for nights once, the result of a conspiracy between a motorway accident (not mine) and overly optimistic timekeeping. It feels much worse to be late to relieve a colleague who has just worked fourteen hours than it feels to be late in the morning.

Some nights the hospital is calm: the ED not too busy, the patients on the wards stable, the emergency bells quiet. Some nights it is in a frenzy: ED is chocka, the patients on the wards are deteriorating, and there are multiple emergency calls happening all over the hospital. You can somehow feel that energy as soon as you walk in the door.

I get a blank piece of paper from the office, which I will fill up with my to-do list for the night, and make my way to handover. Some busier departments start their night shift with a formal handover meeting, with a night team of a few house officers and registrars taking over from the long-day doctors. For others, the handover is finding the long-day doctor on the ward and writing down any outstanding blood tests and scans to be reviewed once results are available, patients who have been sick in the evening shift and what was done for them, and taking the on-call phone and emergency pager. I wish them a good sleep, and they head home to rest for ten hours before tomorrow starts.

I check Task Manager, where nurses put up non-urgent house officer tasks. There are always some simple jobs I can do quickly to make the workload feel smaller — high blood sugars that might need extra insulin, and patients who might die overnight and need to be sighted. Anyone who wants a sleeping tablet gets it: sleeping in hospital is difficult and sleep deprivation doesn't make anyone feel better. Anyone who wants a laxative gets it, although why this is so often requested on the night shift is one of medicine's greatest mysteries.

Once the insulin, sleeping tablets and laxatives are under control, I make a prioritised list of patients who sound like they need an in-person review. Chest pain gets seen fast, because it could represent a heart attack or a blood clot in the lungs. Shortness of breath gets seen fast, especially when it is new or severe. A new fever with other abnormal vital signs like a fast heart rate gets seen fast, because the patient could be newly septic, and will need blood cultures and antibiotics. A review for 'only 500 ml oral intake this shift — consider IV fluids' might get seen eventually.

By the time I have cleared the urgent tasks it is usually close to midnight and most of the patients are asleep. I work through the non-urgent tasks — often just checking that the nurse is happy for the task in question to be dealt with by the daytime staff. I'm not in the business of waking someone up to review their mild earache, and generally think that if the problem isn't one you would go to the After Hours for at midnight, it can wait until morning.

When you're working in a department that has a whole team of night doctors, or when you know the nurses on your ward well, the lulls in a night shift can be a time for gossiping in hushed tones. This is probably one of the nicest things about doing nights: it feels a little bit like being a kid at a sleepover, staying awake talking and giggling until morning. You can start a set of night shifts having barely met, and finish them as friends. Nights are also the time when the nurses' stations have the best snacks. You can usually scrounge up some lollies, and sometimes even pizza.

In smaller departments where there is only one house officer and one reg overnight, nights can be pretty lonely. If the wards are quiet, I might go to ED to help the registrar admit new patients. If ED is quiet, I might get some sleep.

In theory, hospitals provide sleeping facilities for junior doctors. The two beds at Middlemore are located just off the junior doctors' lounge, a cold and drab prefab far away from most hospital wards. If those beds are taken, the only other options are two ancient couches covered in crumbs. No thanks. Some nights I sleep in the doctor's office on the ward, borrowing a pillow and a couple of blankets and curling up on the floor under a desk. On really quiet nights I sleep in one of the clinic rooms downstairs, unused at night except by savvy (and sleepy) junior doctors. The hard examination tables are only slightly more comfortable than the office floor.

Some nights I get three or four hours of broken sleep, putting my phone on loud and setting my alarm every hour to check Task Manager. Some nights are busy enough that I don't even try to sleep. Being woken every ten minutes makes you infinitely more tired than just staying awake. On those nights I make myself a Milo and catch up on paperwork in between phone calls.

On the worst nights I am on my feet with sick patients or at emergency calls the entire night. These are the nights of the patient whose medication is making their blood sugar dangerously low, but who keeps pulling out the IV line we are using to give life-saving sugar replacement. These are the nights where the number of simultaneous emergency calls is exactly equal to the number of doctors on shift, meaning that the registrars can only stop by to give some brief instructions before leaving me and the nurses to carry them out.

Looking after sick people overnight is hard because you are on your own, and because your brain doesn't really work as well on nights as it does during daylight hours. The fatigue makes everything a bit fuzzy, and you have to think very hard to avoid making stupid mistakes. One night, a nurse had to gently point out to me that 0.18 per cent sodium chloride did not in fact have more sodium in it than 0.9 per cent. Worse still, it took me several minutes of counting on my fingers and playing on my calculator until I realised where I had gone wrong.

Around 6.30 a.m. the day shift starts to arrive. I always find the end to the quiet solitude of the night slightly disorienting, although of course very welcome. The nurses have their handover at seven, after which a few extra keen or over-caffeinated nurses will call, wanting me to tick things off their list of outstanding problems for their patient. I chart fluids, pain relief or laxatives. For anything more involved, I remind them (gently, if I can manage it) that the patient's regular team will be there for the day shift in a few minutes.

After handover, it is back to the changing room to get out of my dirty scrubs. On night shifts I usually treat myself by taking home a fresh pair that I can wear back into work that evening, giving me an extra five minutes to stare into space and dread coming in.

The twenty-minute drive home stands between me and my bed. I blast the air conditioning on cold to stay awake, play loud music and make animated facial expressions as I sing along. I must look completely bizarre, but better to look unhinged than to drift off behind the wheel.

Charlie welcomes me home after night shifts like a returning hero. When I am on nights she is always even sorrier for me than I am sorry for myself. She makes me a cooked breakfast, and we eat together before I shuffle off to bed where she has shut the blinds for me, turned down the covers and put a glass of water on the bedside table.

I've been a terrible sleeper for my entire life, having suffered from bouts of insomnia since childhood, and even when my insomnia isn't too bad I only tend to get six hours of sleep each night. By some miracle, I do not have this problem after a night shift. While many of my colleagues can only manage four or five hours, I am a prodigious day-sleeper, and am in the land of nod for a full eight hours as soon as my head hits the pillow. Even so, I always wake up a tiny bit nauseated, and not really refreshed.

I get up, splash my face with some cold water, and take a shower. I stand there for twenty minutes, just staring into space as the warm water runs down my back. Charlie makes dinner and I eat it, fighting against the nausea. I drink my plunger of coffee and get into my clean scrubs. I am only moderately sloppy on day shifts, but on nights all pretence of grooming goes out the window. Messy hair is pulled into a messy bun. I wear a cosy old hoodie over my scrubs, and my warmest woolly socks inside my Crocs. On occasion, I have opted for a crop top instead of a proper bra. The indignity of having to be awake at 4 a.m. is bad enough without also having to contend with underwire.

The first night is the worst for me. That night, I have already been awake all day and I am exhausted, my body and brain not yet accustomed to being awake all night. By the second night I am in a rhythm of sorts, and by the third night the end is in sight.

After the last night shift, all the doctors from the nights team go out for breakfast together, and perhaps a coffee or even a cocktail. We sit in the camaraderie of night shifts for a little longer, and laugh at our new inside jokes. Then we wish one another a good sleep, and head home for our three days off.

CHAPTER 22

Surgery

MY FINAL ROTATION as a first year was in general surgery. I was back on a team with Gaby, working for two upper-gastrointestinal surgeons specialising in problems with the oesophagus, stomach, liver, pancreas and gallbladder.

Some of the sickest patients on general surgery wards are those with upper-GI problems. The pancreas in particular is a formidable foe. Best known for making hormones that are released into the blood to metabolise sugar, it also makes enzymes that are released into our digestive tract to help break down food. When the pancreas is damaged or inflamed, these enzymes can digest us instead. A common saying among surgeons is 'Don't fuck with the pancreas.'

Like most upper-GI surgeons, our bosses were meticulous. They worked hard and held themselves to high standards, and expected the same from their team. Being perfectionists ourselves, this suited both Gaby and me just fine. We were also blessed with very supportive registrars, who always had a handle on what needed to be done for our complex patients, and were happy to answer our questions.

In my first few years of medical school I had always told people I wanted to be a surgeon. After all those years of watching *Grey's*, I figured I knew roughly what to expect. Performing your first surgery in the 'OR' on your very first day, in front of a peanut gallery of other doctors who apparently have nothing better to do than watch nervous interns perform appendectomies. Calling it an 'appendectomy'. Multi-traumas where junior doctors drill burr holes in the bones of a patient's skull with a power drill to save their life. Bombs in body cavities.

Even aside from the absence of compelling, 45-minute patient story arcs, the reality of surgery is nothing like what I had imagined. The operating theatre, just called 'theatre', is the most controlled environment in the hospital. As a new student visiting theatre for the first time you are under the eagle eyes of the theatre nurses, ready to tell you off if you touch anything or get in the way. This isn't entirely because they hate students (although some of them do seem to take a good deal of pleasure in taking us down a peg) — keeping the operating theatre organised and most importantly sterile is literally a matter of life or death.

I am more nervous performing a surgical scrub than I have ever been putting in an IV line or even stitching a wound in ED. First, you open your cleaning sponge, which is doused in iodine or chlorhexidine and has a nail pick and nail brush attached. You use the pick to clean under your nails, and then discard it. At some hospitals you get in trouble if you don't put the pick into the sharps' bin. At others, it just goes into the rubbish.

Next, you use the brush to scrub your nails, hands and forearms, all the way to the elbows. You have to take care not to accidentally touch the taps or soap dispensers while you are scrubbing, or you start again from scratch. Next, depending on who you ask, you either rinse off the solution and wash again twice over, or simply leave the solution in contact with your skin for a full three minutes to allow the antiseptic to kill any bacteria. You wash your hands and arms with water, letting the water run down your arms from your hands to your elbows, from the cleanest to the dirtiest point. You remember not to shake your hands and risk contamination with water from further up your arms, or you start again from scratch.

You walk over to the table where your sterile gown and gloves have been prepared. You don't touch anything non-sterile, nor does any non-sterile part of you touch the table, or you start again from scratch. You dry your hands one at a time with the sterile paper towels that are part of the gown pack, which you throw into the bin after using. You pick up your folded surgical gown and step back so you are well clear of the table before giving it a little shake to let it fall open. You don't let it touch anything, or you start again from scratch.

You slip your arms into the gown, and step back to the table to put your gloves on while your hands are still completely covered by your sleeves, using a technique called 'closed gloving' which I have never quite mastered. A circulating nurse will come over to secure your gown at the back of your neck and at your waist. The final step of securing the gown is a second tie around the waist, which keeps the gown closed. This tie has a piece of cardboard attached, which you hand to an assistant who holds it still while you spin around to close the gown. The piece of cardboard pulls away and you secure the ties.

Once you are scrubbed, you are considered sterile 'from boobs to pubes'. You have to be careful not to touch anything non-sterile, including your own body outside of the sterile area. You clasp your gloved hands in front of you or hold them across your abdomen, to remind you not to touch anything. You have to stay aware of your surroundings at all times to avoid touching anything that will break sterility. This means carefully squeezing past pieces of equipment to get to the correct side of the operating table. It also means that if your glasses slip down your nose you leave them alone, or bravely ask a circulating nurse to push them back up. If a bead of sweat rolls down your forehead into your eye, you let it stay there.

Every operation starts with a 'sign in' while the patient is still awake, to confirm their identity, the operation they are expecting to have, what side they are expecting to have it on, and any allergies. Once the patient is asleep, there is a 'time out' before knife to skin. The person leading the time out follows a checklist printed on the wall of every operating theatre. Shortened checklists are available for emergency operations that need to happen so fast that the normal time-out process is not possible, such as caesareans when the baby's life is at risk. There is a final confirmation of the patient's name, the intended procedure including the site and side, plans for antibiotics to prevent infection and any measures to prevent blood clots, how much blood loss is expected, and whether there are any critical or non-routine steps in the operation. Finally, every person in the room introduces themself by their name and role. Only then can the operation begin.

The operations themselves are much more mundane than television had led me to believe. Three of the most common operations I saw as a student were I&Ds (incision and drainage, cutting open an abscess and draining out the pus), laparoscopic appendicectomies (as we call them here), and 'lap choles' (laparoscopic cholecystectomies, keyhole surgery to remove the gallbladder).

As a medical student, you sometimes get the job of holding and pointing the camera on a stick that goes inside the abdomen to show the surgeon what they're operating on during keyhole surgery. I was so excited the first time I got to do this. My excitement was quickly replaced by a steely determination not to burst into tears until I could do so without my tears falling onto the sterile field. The registrar who was operating wasn't particularly confident performing the procedure, and also wasn't the best communicator. Although it was my first time, he expected me to know where to point the camera without explaining, and grumbled and sighed when I got it wrong. A few minutes in, out of sheer frustration at my incompetence, the consultant scrubbed in to hold the camera, and told me to scrub out and watch. The rest of the operation was peppered with his sarcastic commentary: 'See, Izzy, it helps if the camera is actually pointing at where he is trying to operate.'

Fortunately, being a surgical house officer is not quite like being a surgical medical student. Our job as house officers is to take care of things on the ward while the surgeons are off doing surgery, and there is rarely a need, or indeed an opportunity, for us to be in the operating theatre. When we do go, the staff are much nicer to us than they are to medical students. Even the grumpiest surgeons are generally pretty kind to house officers. We are senior enough to be useful, but not so senior that they want to take us down a peg.

Some consultants can be pretty hard on registrars. The registrars are committed to their specialty, and while the good consultants feel responsible for nurturing them as they grow their knowledge and skills, others see it more as a responsibility to kick them into shape. They grill them at handover in front of everyone, nitpick their case presentations and management plans, and an awful minority even yell at them in front of patients.

The thing about teaching by humiliation is that you teach two lessons. Your junior learns the information you grilled them about, but they also learn the kind of doctor and boss they don't want to become. Or they become just like you, and turn into the type of senior doctor who romanticises the struggle they went through during their training, and complains that juniors are soft these days any time a change is made that improves our working conditions. They worked a hundred-hour week for ten years and got four hours' sleep a night and look how they turned out!

The bullies are in a minority now, I think, but they are still tolerated, and their behaviour goes mostly without consequence. Their identities are an open secret, and if you tell another doctor, 'There was a really mean consultant in A Particular Specialty at A Particular Hospital,' they will usually know exactly who you mean. Some consultants will periodically be banned from having students because there are so many complaints, but these bans never seem to last long.

I have been fortunate. All through medical school and my time as a doctor I have accidentally found my way onto 'the good team' that everyone wants to be on. My bosses have been kind, supportive and appreciative when I do a good job. My efforts have been rewarded in coffees and team dinners, and the one or two mistakes I have been told off badly for were quickly forgotten. My stupid questions have usually been answered kindly.

On the odd occasion when I have felt unfairly told off, or have seen a registrar grilled particularly cruelly, I have had excellent colleagues to bitch about it with afterwards. Sam is an A+ complaining buddy, and his exclamations of 'Oh my god, sis, I know!' were punctuation for the more frustrating parts of the job. Gaby can roll her eyes with more venom than anyone else I've met. Brittany is usually gentle and positive, and when she says, 'Yeah, it's not the best,' it hits as hard as it would if someone else swore. It's nice to be part of a team.

CHAPTER 23:

Christmas Eve

IT WAS CHRISTMAS Eve. The day started like any other. I woke up at 5.30, threw on comfy clothes and ordered my morning latte from the cafe at the petrol station. I had worked until 10 p.m. the night before and I was absolutely wrecked, so I treated myself to a pastry for breakfast instead of my glovebox muesli bar.

The motorway was quiet that early, and I arrived at work around six and got changed into scrubs. I printed the list of patients and set to work looking up vital signs, blood-test results, and the times for any scans that had been booked by the doctor who admitted them. I also prepared the ward-round notes using a printed template. A surgical ward round goes so fast that on busy days we found that easier.

My team was post-acute. It had been a particularly awful acute day, with a lot of sad cases and very sick people who didn't yet have firm diagnoses.

General surgery is a specialty that relies fairly heavily on scans to make a diagnosis. Some areas of medicine deal with illnesses that can be diagnosed mostly with blood tests. Some areas deal with illnesses that can be diagnosed clinically, just based on signs and symptoms. General surgery is not like that. Experienced doctors can have a good guess at what might be going on in a sick person with abdominal pain, but they will still be surprised by scan results fairly often. Before doctors routinely used imaging to confirm appendicitis, there were a fair few operations that removed a normal appendix.

Scanning slots in the radiology department are one of the most precious and contested resources at a busy hospital. The radiologists have the unenviable job of telling people like me, whose bosses have asked them to call and arrange an urgent scan, that there is no way on God's green earth that my stable patient with barely elevated inflammatory markers is getting a CT today.

Christmas was a four-day weekend, and on weekends the hospital operates with a skeleton staff. Only urgent scans get done, and even if a scan goes ahead, the other departments who might need to be called in to treat the problem once it is diagnosed are all on holiday. As a result, every junior doctor in the hospital on Christmas Eve was doing their best to sell their patient as the sickest one, the one who needed the scan more urgently than the rest.

I had three patients who needed ultrasound scans of their gallbladder and liver on Christmas Eve. After we saw the first of these, my boss was worried enough to ask me to get straight on the phone and beg for an urgent slot, even though we were still on the ward round. I called the radiologist, whose phone had been ringing all morning and who already had almost no ultrasound slots left. When he heard about the patient's blood results and vital signs he was worried too, and rearranged the day to give us an earlier scan.

The second patient wasn't as sick as the first, but if our

suspicions about her diagnosis were correct, she had the potential to deteriorate fast. The radiologist offered me an afternoon scan, one of the last ones available, which I gratefully accepted.

When we got to the third patient, the boss thought he probably had the same problem as the second patient, although his blood results were slightly worse. This time the radiologist sighed. 'Even if we find a stone, do you really think gastro would ERCP him over the long weekend?'

At this point I did what all good house officers do when they're stuck, and name-dropped my consultant. 'Mr Boss is really worried, and he personally asked me to call and try to get a scan today.'

I don't know how, but he managed to find space for all three patients. Around lunchtime, the first patient's ultrasound report came back. There was no evidence of a stone obstructing his bile duct, and the scan hadn't shown a problem with the gallbladder either. It didn't fit with what we were seeing clinically, so my boss asked me to order a specialised MRI scan of the upper abdomen, called an MRCP. I crawled back to the radiologist to beg for one last scan.

The MRI technician and radiologist stayed late to squeeze my patient in, the last case of the day. When he got to the scanner he was delirious and couldn't stay still. Usually the MRI staff don't have time to troubleshoot something like that and have to send the patient back to the ward, but they knew how worried we were about this man, so they called me and said that if I could sedate him they would still do the scan. I hurried down and gave him a tiny dose of IV sedation, which made him relaxed and sleepy, and then the scan proceeded without further hitch.

It was 5 p.m. by this point, an hour after my shift technically finished, but I still had a few hours of work left to do. I headed back upstairs to the ward, then realised I had left my to-do list in the MRI room. I left my phone on the desk in the doctors' office and went back down to MRI.

When I got there, the radiologist who was reporting the scan flagged me down. 'I was just trying to call you. Your team was right about how sick this patient is. Perforated gallbladder. Tomorrow would have been too late.'

The stressful day caught up with me, and I thanked him and burst into relieved and frightened tears.

When I got back upstairs to my phone, I had missed a text from my senior reg, asking if I was still at the hospital. I called him, and as soon as he could safely pull over to let his partner drive, we formulated a plan. The patient needed the interventional radiologist to insert a cholecystostomy tube to drain the infected fluid from the burst gallbladder. He had dementia and a superimposed delirium, and didn't have the capacity to consent, so I also needed to find the surgical registrar to sign a 'consent without capacity' form on my boss's behalf.

It was 5.30 p.m. on Christmas Eve and the interventional radiologist had gone home. I called him and explained the situation, and the fact that we had only just found out the diagnosis after hours. He agreed to come back in, and would be there in about twenty minutes.

I pre-filled the consent form for the on-call surgical registrar to sign, then went to explain to the patient's wife and daughter what the diagnosis was, and the plan. I tried to convey how serious the problem was, while also reassuring them that we were doing everything we could. I told them I only had a few minutes, and I wished I could talk for longer but I needed to organise treatment urgently. I explained how the procedure would work, and some of the risks (bleeding, puncturing something unintentionally, and the need for further procedures). His wife spoke English as a second language and some of the medical words were lost on her, but his daughter interpreted. They were appreciative of our care, and wanted whatever we thought was the best treatment option.

My day still had no end in sight, but I had never seen this procedure done so I went down to interventional radiology to watch on the screen in the radiographer's room. The whole team there had been called back from home: a radiographer, two nurses and the radiologist. If they were annoyed that we had interrupted their Christmas Eve plans with their families, they didn't show it. The whole thing only took a few minutes. A drain went in and the pus was drained. The patient was sent back to the ward. I breathed for the first time in an hour.

All day, in between the times I was organising scans, all manner of chaos had been unfolding. One patient was in acute kidney failure, with his level of potassium getting high enough that we needed to take action or it could send his heart into a deadly rhythm. Two patients had a new diagnosis of cancer, shit news to get at any time, but especially on Christmas Eve.

An older man had been fully treated for the problem he was admitted with, but a blood test incidentally showed that the effect of his blood thinner was five times greater than it should have been. This put him at high risk of bleeding, including bleeding into his brain. Unfortunately, this result was only noticed after he had been told he could go home. He was still on the premises, but his daughter was already driving in to pick him up and he didn't want to put her out by staying for treatment, so he left before I could convince him to stay.

I called him several times, and called his daughter, explaining the situation. When I'm really worried about a patient, I call from my personal phone. If you get a missed call from the generic hospital number you have no way of calling back the person trying to contact you, but a missed call from a mobile gives you the option to text or call back.

His daughter was stressed out. She was juggling childcare and last-minute Christmas shopping, and couldn't understand why we had sent her dad home if he actually needed to be in hospital. I apologised, agreed with her that it shouldn't have happened, listened as she vented both her justified frustration at the hospital and the general frustrations of the stressful Christmas period in my direction. I explained why I was so worried about her dad: when the action of blood thinners is too great, patients are at risk for bleeding, including a brain bleed. She agreed to bring him back to the hospital.

I spoke to a Genl Med consultant, who advised me what needed to be done. He specified the dose of antidote needed to partially reverse the blood thinner so that it still had some effect (which the patient needed). It was the day before a four-day weekend, and most of the community labs and pharmacies had closures or reduced hours over Christmas. He would need to be seen by one of the Gen Med teams each day over the weekend to get his levels rechecked, and get more antidote if needed. I sent a referral through to ED so that the triage nurse knew we were expecting this patient, and would send him straight through to the Gen Med doctors.

Many hours later his daughter called me back. She had been busy earlier, but now they were nearly at the hospital and she was hoping I could organise for them to bypass ED. That wasn't possible, and I told her so. She wasn't too pleased to hear this. She uttered a few choice words and asked what would happen if they just went home. With all the composure I could muster four hours after my rostered finish time, I told her I thought that would be a mistake. Her dad needed care, and the hospital had procedures in place during the pandemic that meant they would need to go through screening before coming to the Medical Assessment Unit. Reluctantly, she agreed.

A few minutes later the patient himself called me to tell me they were in the Medical Assessment Unit. I came down to see which doctors were on that evening, hoping to beg one of them for a favour. One of the other first-year house officers, who I knew a little bit and who lived with Brittany, was working in MAU that evening. She was happy to see my patient next, and I went to tell the patient and his daughter that we had a plan figured out and that they would be seen soon. The daughter was very apologetic about the conversation earlier. She told me she was glad her dad was going to get the care he needed, and wished me a happy Christmas.

It was 8 p.m. and my to-do list was diminishing only slightly faster than my will to live. I had one more discharge to do — someone who the team had decided late could go home if she was feeling up to it. She was over the moon; I did her discharge paperwork and a prescription for strong pain relief and sent her on her way. The last job of the day was to write weekend plans for the patients still in hospital.

The doctors working the weekend are responsible for all the patients on the wards, not just their own team. Weekends are busy, with urgent tasks and sick patients taking priority. A weekend plan is made by the team that usually looks after a patient, to help out their busy colleagues. It is a summary of the patient's relevant medical history and current problems, including the management we are expecting to continue over the weekend, and suggestions for troubleshooting if something goes wrong.

I wrote out the weekend plans, and added the patients I was particularly worried about to our handover board so that everyone coming on shift would be aware of them. I finished at 10 p.m. for the second day in a row, and congratulated myself on having booked my flight home for first thing Christmas morning, rather than after work on Christmas Eve.

I had been meaning to get a COVID swab earlier that day but had barely had a free moment to pee, let alone walk to the building where the swabs were done. One of my favourite nurses swabbed me instead, and I walked the sample to the lab. I got out of my scrubs, drove home while indulging in a

Vital Signs

little motorway cry, packed a bag for my time away, and set a 4 a.m. alarm. I slept the whole shuttle ride to the airport, and the whole flight to Christchurch, before picking up the car and my sisters and driving us the three hours to Reefton where the family was having Christmas.

Reefton is where my grandparents Daisy and Bill live, and since I was little it has been my favourite holiday destination. I sleep in a spare room still decorated with posters from my aunties' teenage years in the eighties, and take walks by the Inangahua River in crisp air that smells of coal smoke. Daisy does my backlog of laundry, offers me a hot drink every few hours, cooks hearty meals and challenges me to game after game of Bananagrams. Bill sits in a La-Z-Boy reading books or watching westerns, and offering cheeky commentary and controversial opinions to wind us up.

Sometimes we go to the tearooms for a coffee, and they introduce me proudly to people we run into on the main street. We browse the shops, and Daisy always shows off a tote bag I embroidered for her as a present. On warm days we eat dinner outside at their faded plastic picnic table, beside Daisy's chrysanthemums. Their simple Summerhill Stone house is my favourite place on earth.

On Christmas Day, as I pulled into their driveway, I relaxed for the first time in 24 hours. I barely made it through lunch before retreating to the room full of eighties posters for a three-hour nap.

CHAPTER 243

A wedding and a funeral

ONCE, IN A small town hospital where everyone knew everyone's business, I helped to set up a hospital wedding.

The groom's mum was an inpatient on the medical ward. She was a patient well known to the staff after months of coming in and out for chemotherapy, complications and symptom management. She and her family had known for a long while that she was going to die of her cancer, and they knew now that it would be pretty soon. They had organised their wedding as early as possible so that she could be there.

Unfortunately, her health had taken a turn and it didn't look likely she would make it to the weekend. She certainly wouldn't be well enough to leave the hospital. They decided to have a small wedding ceremony that afternoon in the hospital chapel, in advance of their reception that weekend.

The doctors, nurses and a pharmacist on the ward where she was being cared for put their heads together and hatched a plan to make their wedding day as special as possible. The pharmacist was a friend of mine, and when she told me what they were planning I knew I had to help. One of the junior doctors and I went on our lunch break to The Warehouse and to the local supermarket. We picked up a bouquet of fresh flowers, bunting, garlands, balloons in pretty pastel colours, and fairy lights. We brought extra fairy lights and lamps from home, and I picked an enormous pile of flowers and foliage from the hospital garden. Other staff in the hospital caught wind of what was going on and brought bunches of flowers and extra decorations. Then we set to work turning the hospital chapel into a wedding venue.

It was a plain and unassuming little room, save for a huge stained-glass window behind the wooden altar. We framed the window with an arch of greenery, flowers and fairy lights. Bunting and a balloon garland adorned the walls, and we arranged as many lamps as we could find around the room to give a glowing light nicer than the fluorescent overheads. We made a big floral arrangement on the altar with fern leaves and flowers. We arranged the chairs with an aisle down the middle, and a big open space at the back where the groom's mum could be brought in on her hospital bed.

Someone had thought of borrowing a few tiny chairs from the Children's Ward for the young kids who were attending, and we seated them right at the front. One of the doctors who had recently married had a nice version of Pachelbel's 'Canon in D' downloaded on her laptop, and she gave it to the family to play while the bride walked in. We all went home and left them to spend a bittersweet evening together as a family, celebrating the couple's love for each other, and their love for his mum.

A wedding and a funeral

It was in that same small town where I went to my first (and so far only) patient funeral. Callum was only four, sick for most of his life with a mysterious illness that would only be diagnosed after he died. It caused progressive weakness and developmental delay. He had been assigned as my 'long case' for paediatrics at the start of the year, so my classmate Jimi and I spent a fair bit of time with Callum and his mum, Sarah.

Sarah was a force of nature. She kept every piece of paper the hospital ever gave her, every discharge summary, copies of every X-ray, even Callum's first hospital wristband. These were pasted in unlined exercise books, along with treasures like artworks that Callum had made, and the words to his favourite songs. Everything was in yellow, his favourite colour. The first day we went to visit her at home for our assignment, she gave us the books to read through. There were four of them and we read every page.

I was on placement in the Emergency Department when Callum came in with severe pneumonia. The small amount of food and drink he took orally (rather than into his feeding tube) seemed to be getting into his lungs and, on top of that, his breathing muscles were becoming so weak that he couldn't effectively cough to clear his normal phlegm.

We treated the pneumonia, but his breathing still worsened. He was in hospital with his breathing supported, but he continued to deteriorate.

I was on a placement an hour away when I got the call that he wasn't expected to survive the weekend. That was on a Friday afternoon. I drove back to see Sarah, and to say goodbye to Callum. I expected her to be a wreck, but I suppose I should have known she would be holding it together. She smiled and joked with me, grateful, I think, for a momentary distraction from her grief.

'When anyone from my life visits, I end up being the one comforting them,' she observed.

Vital Signs

Callum wasn't conscious by this point. He had soft toys under his feet to prevent pressure areas on the heels. He looked peaceful, the morphine ensuring he didn't feel breathless and wasn't in any pain.

I came back to visit the following morning. I asked Sarah if there was anything I could do for her. She told me she wanted more doctors and medical students to know about Callum. I told her I would do my best. I gave Callum a little pat on the top of his foot, and said, 'See you later, mate.'

I had an essay due, so I went to the library to write about his pneumonia. He had looked deceptively well when he came in, because his muscles were too weak to do the usual increased work of breathing that tells us when someone's lungs are struggling. I wrote about this, and about how guidelines for care of children with neuromuscular conditions stress the importance of listening to their caregivers, whose idea of 'normal' is specific to this particular child, rather than healthy children in general.

I went back after dinner to check on Callum. When I arrived at the Children's Ward, the nurse was someone I hadn't met before. She asked who I was, and what I was doing there.

'I'm Izzy, one of the medical students. I'm just popping in on Callum.'

She gave me a sympathetic look, led me into the staff tearoom, and shut the door.

'I'm sorry, Callum passed. About half an hour ago. Sarah's in there with him now.'

'Oh. Thank you for letting me know.'

I walked back to the library, utterly numb.

His funeral was on Wednesday. Jimi and I sat in the back of the packed funeral home, next to Callum's GP, who we knew well, and one of the ED doctors from the hospital. A big group of nurses from the Children's Ward sat a few rows ahead, most of them weeping openly. Family, friends and his preschool teacher stood up to speak. Callum had touched a lot of hearts in his short life.

We sang his favourite song, 'Morningtown Ride'. His family lit candles, one for each year of his life. Just four candles. The tears that had been prickling behind my eyes spilled over then. At the end of the service we formed a double line like school kids, to lay flowers in the back of a yellow Tonka truck and wish Sarah well. The two doctors lined up in front of Jimi and me. I was grateful to see them modelling how to be when your chest is bursting, filled by air heavy with a grief that isn't really yours.

I think that is part of what dulls the sadness of patient deaths over time: the belief that it isn't your place to feel so sad about someone who, while *a* person, isn't *your* person.

I cried a lot about Callum though, at home. I still think about him a lot, and about Sarah too. I think about how inconsequential most four-year periods of my life have been, filled with loves and feuds that meant everything to me at the time but that I can barely remember a few years later. Sarah is about the same age as me, and yet four years of her life contained the entirety of his. I don't know how you recover from something like that. I don't know if you do.

We visited her once more, when we had finished our rural year and were getting ready to move back to our home campuses. We drank tea in her lounge and made small talk, and asked how she was, and meant it. She cried talking about how quiet life felt with him gone, and how she didn't know what she would do with the mobility van now that she didn't have his wheelchair to move. I gave her a copy of *The BFG*, which Roald Dahl had dedicated to his daughter who died of measles. She cried again, and hugged us goodbye.

CHAPTER 25:

Endings

IN THE LAST week of our first year, all our patients were getting sicker. Gaby and I had planned to spend that week getting all of our discharges prepped and handover documents organised for the new house officers taking over the team. Instead, it felt like we spent the whole week in 777 emergency calls for three of our long stayers, and walking the delicate line between dehydrating them and putting them into fluid overload.

Friday was our last team meeting. I wasn't rostered to be there because I was starting nights that evening, but I came in to say goodbye. An unspoken rule for medical students was that you should bring baking to say thank you to the ward staff and your medical team on the last day of your run, and many of us continued this as house officers. I specialise in cheese scones, while Gaby makes a mean brownie. The bosses and registrars thanked us for all our hard work on the team, and wished us the best for our next rotations. I was moving to another hospital to do obstetrics and gynaecology, one of the areas of medicine I like the most, while future surgeon Gaby was staying at Middlemore to do surgical relief.

I gave Gaby a hug goodbye, and got a little choked up realising that I'd had my last day as her offsider. She had been my closest colleague and best work friend for a full six months, and now we wouldn't even be working in the same hospital. I think we will be friends forever, but I know that once you aren't working together it's never really the same.

The night shifts that weekend were the quietest I've had. Even so, the knowledge that those were my last few hours at Middlemore meant I couldn't sleep at all, and when there were no patients to see I caught up on the handover preparation that we had been too busy to do during the week. When that was done, I sat in the stillness and dark and quiet of a hospital that had come to feel like home.

The team had a busy post-acute day on Monday morning, and I showed the new house officers how to prep the list of new patients to be seen. Soon, the room was filling up with strangers and it was time for handover. My job was done. I changed out of my scrubs, handed in my ID card and my parking card, ordered one last coffee from Elixir, and waved goodbye to the security guard as I walked out of my first year as doctor, and into the sunshine.

Finishing up that first year felt like another graduation of sorts. No longer brand new, I was now a doctor with general registration, with a whole year in the trenches at one of the busiest hospitals in the country.

I didn't have much time to reflect on it, as I started a busy new rotation straight away, and a few weeks later New Zealand's Omicron outbreak took off. Then I was truly a pandemic doctor for the first time. I learned the ropes of the new rotation (and wrote the first draft of this book) while our case numbers were in the tens of thousands, and discovered a level of exhaustion unlike anything I had previously known. With many of our colleagues falling sick we were inundated with requests to pick up extra shifts. Thankfully, doctors and nurses from services not deemed 'mission critical' were redeployed to the hospitals, which helped a lot. I learned how to assess COVID patients for their risk of deterioration, who needed steroids, and how to decide which pregnant COVID patients needed blood thinners to prevent clots.

On my first day as a doctor I was equal parts eager and terrified, sick of being a student but not feeling at all ready to be a doctor. You adapt. Like a root-bound pot finally replanted, I have grown to fit my new job, and even to work through a pandemic. The everyday tasks that once filled me with dread have now become routine. In time, I will outgrow them. A friend and fellow house officer once said she thought that people didn't step up because they felt ready to be a registrar, but because they felt so sick of being a house officer.

In my early twenties, before I decided to go to medical school, I had a bit of a quarter-life crisis about what to be when I grew up. I was young enough that most options were available to me (although I'd sadly missed the window to be an Olympic figure skater), but old enough that other people my age were finishing degrees and starting careers, and I had no idea what I wanted to do. I enjoyed my job at Parliament but knew that I didn't want to be an executive assistant forever. I was so relieved when I decided to go to medical school. The decision was made, and I knew what I was going to be: a doctor.

I didn't really know any doctors before I went to medical school. Six years of study sounded like an awfully long time, and I don't think I really understood that those six years were only the beginning. I didn't realise that 'a doctor' was only really the start of a decision about what to do with my life.

I've been a doctor for a year now, and I still don't really know what I want to be when I grow up. I enjoy most areas of medicine, and so far the epiphany I've been waiting for hasn't come. Or perhaps it's more accurate to say that I have had the epiphany many times over, as I have fallen in love with most of the specialities I've tried. I enjoy surgery, but I also enjoy making the thorough and meticulous problem lists they have in Gen Med. I love obstetrics, but I don't know if I want to commit to doing caesareans at 3 a.m. for the rest of my working life. I love hospitals, but I also think 'GP-land' is the most important part of medicine, and that walking alongside patients for decades through their life's ups and downs is the most sacred form of doctoring.

My training journey is only just beginning. I have at least another year as a house officer before I can start a more specialised job as a registrar, and many more years of apprenticing, studying and sitting gruelling exams in that field before I am a fully qualified specialist.

Medical school exams are a hassle. They're stressful, tiring and often examine obscure parts of the curriculum that weren't highlighted when the subjects were taught. They also come with a guaranteed short study break, and almost all students pass.

Doctor exams are a different beast. These exams cost thousands of dollars (fortunately reimbursable by our employers) to attempt. Intelligent, dedicated, hard-working people can spend all their free time studying, every waking hour outside their 60-hour work week for an entire year, and still fail. It would be fair to say I am not looking forward to them.

Exams are just one hurdle doctors take on in order to specialise. Juniors in surgical fields spend their first few years as non-training registrars collecting 'points' for their CVs. You can get them from work experience as a non-trainee (though these expire after a certain time), from preparing relevant research papers and conference presentations, and from completing higher education such as a Masters or PhD relevant to the specialty.

Your bosses give references on standardised forms which are scored in order to numerically rank candidates. The top candidates qualify for an interview, which often attracts a fee just to attend. For the most competitive specialties, such as paediatric surgery and orthopaedics, there are many more people who hope to get a place in training than can ever actually get one. You can apply a limited number of times, and if you don't get a place with any of those applications, you just have to find a new dream.

Non-training registrars work their guts out to try to impress their bosses and get references good enough to earn them a spot on the training programme. Sometimes that can mean six months of biting your tongue while working for a difficult boss. Sometimes it can mean moving around the country collecting experience at hospitals whose consultants are known for getting their juniors into training.

Once you're actually in a training programme, you will probably be required to move at least once or twice, leaving your support system and uprooting your kids if you're lucky enough to already have them. If you don't have kids yet and want them, you'll have to either take time off training to go on parental leave, or risk waiting until after you finish your training and hope that you don't have fertility problems.

Studying for final exams is gruelling and difficult as a single person with no family responsibilities; with children to look after, it is nearly impossible. If you are a couple who are both doctors, as Charlie and I will be, parenting while training really means you have to take it in turns. Both parents can't be at exam crunch time at the same time, not unless the kids have grandparents who are *really* keen to have a second go at raising children.

I didn't know any of this when I went into medicine. I have always liked working, and get a lot of satisfaction from throwing myself into my work, especially when I am doing a job that feels useful to the world. I always figured that the hardest part was going to be the six years at university, because studying was never something I particularly enjoyed. At the start of medical school, those six years felt impossibly long and daunting. I very nearly decided that it was too much study, even for my dream job. I don't think I would have decided to do it if I had known just how much study would still stretch out before me at this point, how much of my life would have to be sacrificed to training. I suppose I'm glad I didn't know.

When I injured my ankle, just before moving to Dunedin to start medical school, I shyly told the English ED doctor I was going to study medicine. She would have been a registrar I guess, probably up to her eyeballs in exam prep. I asked her if she had any advice. She looked at me with dead eyes and said, not in jest, 'Don't do it.'

If I could go back in time, would I listen to her? Probably not. Medicine is hard, but it's also incredible. Sure, there are days and weeks when I come home so bone tired that I can barely string a sentence together, when I have used every bit of emotional capacity on my patients and have none left for me. There are days when I only just make it to my car before the tears spill out. There are days when the weight of the things I've seen and the stories of the patients I've met are so heavy they threaten to smother me. There are days when I feel my newness and my awkwardness so keenly that I have no idea how I can ever hope to be any good at this job.

But then there are days when all I can feel is awe that I get the privilege of doing this job, holding space for people on the worst days of their lives. There are days when I get to see the best that humans can be, the greatest feats of hope and love. There are days sitting in my scrubs in the sunshine that I look at my colleagues and think, 'Yup, these are my people.' There are days when I learn something new that fascinates me, and I light up thinking about getting to learn more about how bodies work for the rest of my life. There are days when I can make a difference, and I get to come home and tell my flatmates that 'I was a good doctor today.'

My boss at Parliament, Russel Norman, was a medical student for four years before he decided to quit and study politics. He decided that the world needed better politicians more than it needed better doctors. In my last few weeks of working for him we were having office drinks, and he told me the only way to change things was upstream, through service design. He believed you couldn't change things on the front line. I still don't agree with him, but I understand what he meant now, more than I did before.

I can spend my whole life working to be a Pākehā doctor who tries to practise in a culturally safe way, and it will make vastly less difference for Māori health overall than a government policy to address the housing crisis, or a treaty settlement that gives back stolen land. But doctors are uniquely placed to advocate for policy changes that will benefit public health. We hold a respected position in society, and our advocacy holds some weight. And even in a world where all the social determinants of health have been addressed and all the upstream interventions have been made, we will still need doctors, and we need them to be good ones. I think I can be one of the good ones. I hope I can.

I don't know if I am trying to convince you, or trying to convince myself. I think medicine is where I need to be right now. I love being a doctor, and I love working directly with patients. I think the health system is made up of good people who are doing the best they can with the resources they have. I also think it could be a lot better, and I believe we can make it better.

I'm sure that when I am a consultant, older and greyer than I am now, I will chuckle and cringe as I look back on these musings, written when I had just turned one in doctor years, still learning to walk really. I haven't seen all that much yet, and I don't know all that much. But I know how it feels at the very start, and I think that will still matter. Every single day my heart and mind are stretched further by this challenging, exhausting and incredible job. Every single day as a doctor takes me further away from the teenage girl who watched Meredith, Cristina, Izzie and George start work on *Grey's Anatomy* and dreamed that one day it could be her.

I hope I make her proud.

ACKNOWLEDGEMENTS

TO MY FAMILY: Daisy, Bill, Michelle, Martin, William, Jemima, Georgina, Harry, Andrew, Anna, Sonya, Alexis, Dave, Josh, Aurelia, and the many cats. I love you all very much. Thank you for your endless love and support, and for your encouragement as I took on the mammoth task of writing this. I'm sorry I am always at the hospital when you call.

To Charlie: thank you for being my person while I lived my first year as a doctor, for spurring me on while I wrote about it, and for your patience in reading draft after draft and giving thoughtful feedback each time. I love you, and I will make all those loads of laundry up to you one day.

To my flatmates at La Roche: thank you for all the coffee, chocolate and encouraging words you gave me while I was writing this. Thanks to Āria Newfield, Paige Edwards and Sophie Dowsett for being three of my very first readers.

To the world's best offsiders, Gaby, Sam, and Brittany: thank you for living this year alongside me, and for agreeing to be part of it on the page. You are wonderful humans and wonderful doctors.

To Emma Espiner and Lauren Spence: thank you for welcoming me to Auckland and for replying whenever I vented in your DMs. To Sashika Samaranayaka: thank you for being my first work friend!

To Wilbur Townsend and Prasanthi Cottingham: thank you for making Auckland feel like home, and for making me honorary aunt to the world's best and cleverest baby.

Thank you to my publisher, Michelle Hurley, for believing that I could write a book long before I believed it myself; to my editor, Tracey Wogan, for understanding what I was trying to say and helping me to make it better; and to Saskia Nicol for the beautiful cover design. Thank you to Leanne McGregor for overseeing the editing and publishing process, to publicist Abba Renshaw, and to the rest of the Allen & Unwin team. Thank you to Emma Neale and Rachel Scott for proofreading.

A huge thank you to Simon Rickit and Rachel Gerber at Meredith Connell for helping me get my head around contracts!

Endless thanks to Sarah for letting me be part of Callum's final days, and letting me tell his story. Thank you to David for graciously letting me tell yours. Thank you to Hermione for letting me borrow your worst days, and for letting me stick around for the best ones. Thank you to Lucy for letting me write about your experiences. Thank you to Julia for opening my eyes to the realities of caring for a loved one at home.

Thank you to Animesh Chatterjee for showing me the kind of doctor I want to be, and for teaching me about loss of hypoxic vasoconstriction. Thank you to Farid Shaba for letting me borrow your acronyms and for all the whiteboard teaching at handover! Thank you to Linda Grady for teaching me clinical skills, and to Ernie for teaching me to drive so patiently.

Thank you to Russel Norman for being an incredible boss, and for not letting me get away with thinking that just 'helping people' on the front line is enough. If I can make even half as much good Green change in the world as you have, I will be very proud.

Thanks to David Murdoch and the University of Otago for letting me share the graduation speech and the Oath.

Thank you to the more senior doctors who taught and helped me during my first year, especially Joe O'Connor, Chris Zhang, Stewart Shiu, Jennifer Chieng, Khalid El Kashlan, Nealie Barker, Millie Eddowes, Tyler Campbell, Renus Stowers, Amelia Shin, Katherine Given, Frankie Finch, Thanikk Corattur, Bo Jiang, Tiana Wu, Josh Balhorn, Mark Pang, Clare Hollewand,

Acknowledgements

Waldron Martis, Andy Veale, Lit Yoong, Kurt Wendelborn, Matt Tomlinson, Simon Manners, Alpesh Patel, Suren Senthi, Diana McNeill, Vigna Vignakumar, Yoomi Clarkson, Andrew MacCormick and Jon Morrow.

Thank you to all the other doctors, nurses, pharmacists, allied health workers, ward clerks, healthcare assistants, support staff, orderlies and cleaners at Middlemore Hospital. There are too many of you to name, but you all do incredible work for patients and whānau, and you made Middlemore feel like home.

Finally, thank you to the patients past, present and future who let me walk alongside them for a little while.

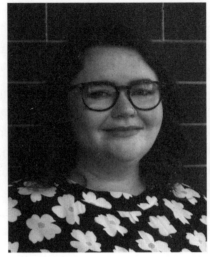

Author photo by Paige Edwards

ABOUT THE AUTHOR

IZZY LOMAX-SAWYERS IS a doctor and a keen writer. She grew up in Westport as the oldest of six feral kids. Along with her MBChB from the University of Otago, she has a BA in Linguistics from Victoria University of Wellington. Her writing has featured in *The New Zealand Herald*, the *Poetry New Zealand Yearbook*, and on the medical humanities blog Corpus.